AF542949

MEDICINE AND INTEGRATION OF FRONTIER TRIBES

Medicine and Integration of Frontier Tribes

The British and After in Arunachal Pradesh

TAJEN DABI

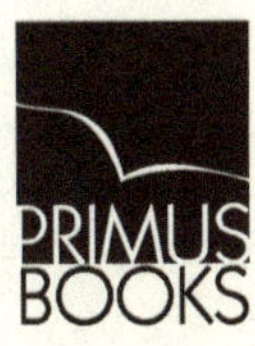

PRIMUS BOOKS
An imprint of Ratna Sagar P. Ltd.
Virat Bhavan
Mukherjee Nagar Commercial Complex
Delhi 110 009

Offices at CHENNAI LUCKNOW
AGRA AHMEDABAD BENGALURU COIMBATORE DEHRADUN GUWAHATI
HYDERABAD JAIPUR JALANDHAR KANPUR KOCHI KOLKATA MADURAI
MUMBAI PATNA RANCHI VARANASI

First published 2023

ISBN: 978-93-5687-046-8 (Hardback)
ISBN: 978-93-5687-044-4 (PoD)

Published by Primus Books

Lasertypeset by Sai Graphic Design
Arakashan Road, Paharganj, New Delhi 110 055

Contents

Abbreviations

APO	Assistant Political Officer
ASA	Assam State Archives, Dispur
AR	Assam Rifles
AS	Assistant Surgeon
CAS	Civil Assistant Surgeon
CS	Civil Surgeon
DC	Deputy Commissioner
DDT	Dichloro Diphenyl Trichloroethane
DHS	Director of Health Services, NEFA
DIPR	Directorate of Information and Public Relations, Government of Arunachal Pradesh (GoAP)
DMO	District Medical Officer
EIC	East India Company
FT	Frontier Tract
HD	Hansen's Disease or Leprosy
ICA	International Council for Archives
IMS	Indian Medical Service
IGCH	Inspector-General of Civil Hospitals, Assam
JCO	Junior Commissioned Officer
MEP	Malaria Eradication Programme
MSL	Metres above Sea Level
NA	Not available
NAI	National Archives of India, New Delhi
NCAER	National Council of Applied Economic Research
NEFT	North-East Frontier Tract
NEFA	North-East Frontier Agency
NMEP	National Malaria Eradication Programme

List of Abbreviations

NSEP	National Smallpox Eradication Programme
PO	Political Officer
SAGAP	State Archives, Government of Arunachal Pradesh, Itanagar
TB	Tuberculosis
UT	Union Territory
VD	Venereal Disease
WBM	Western Biomedicine

Plates, Figures and Tables

Plates

Figure

Tables

Preface

This book focuses on generating a new domain of knowledge within an existing genre of historical research, that is, British colonial interventions in the eastern Himalayas. I owe a lot to Professor Tana Showren, who was my doctoral supervisor. He charged me with pursuing a new theme within the genre of British-tribes relationships and the result is this book which has been chiselled out, with deviations, omissions, and new inputs in the form of two new chapters, from my doctoral work titled 'Development of Healthcare System in Arunachal Pradesh, 1826–1987' submitted to the Rajiv Gandhi University, Itanagar in 2017. Of all people who contributed most to this work, Professor Showren's name must naturally come first. I feel it a privilege to have been mentored by him.

Colleagues, friends, and relatives were resourceful with logistics and timely encouragement. I would like to mention the names of the following people in this regard: Professor Shyam Narayan Singh, Professor Sudhir Kumar Singh, Professor Sarah Hilaly, Professor Ashan Riddi, Dr Tade Sangdo, Professor David R. Syiemlieh, Professor Amrendra Kumar Thakur, Professor Tomo Riba, Professor A.K. Das, Professor Nani Bath, Dr Vandana Upadhaya, Dr Maila Lama, Professor Jumyir Basar, Professor Vinay Srivastav, Dr Mie Dirchi, Dr Atsuko Ibata, Dr Gibji Nimasow, Dr Lijum Noshi, Dr David Gao, Dr Chera Tamak, Ms Kitoholi Zhimo, Mr Mintu Mushahary, Mrs Jarjum Gamlin Ete, Mr Kaling Jerang, Ms Chikap Dabi, Mr Tapak Dabi, Mr Tagam Dabi, Mrs Minya Nyodu Basar, and Mr Tade Dabi (pastor). I humbly record my gratitude to each one of them.

The Indian Council of Historical Research (ICHR), New Delhi, provided travel expenses for visiting archives. I am grateful to the ICHR for the grant. My field-study trips to Bomdila and Tawang in western Arunachal were facilitated and helped by Professor Tana Showren, Ms Konchok Dolma, Mr Namge Tsering, Mr Rinchin Norbu, Mr Dondup Tsering, Mr Tsering Topgey, His Eminence Guru Tulku Rinpoche, Abbot, Gaden Namgyal Lhatse (Tawang Monastery), and Wangdi Lama, monk, Khinmey Monastery, Tawang. Fellow clan members and elders from my native village Nyiga Tari Dabi, Nyiga Tarik Dabi, and Nyiga Kabom Dabi provided me with insights on indigenous rituals and healing systems. Nyib Tama Mindo, shaman, Tadar Nipo, son of late shaman Nyubh Tadar Nyajung, and the all-knowing Nyikok Babin Karlo, folk rhapsodist readily shared their knowledge and experiences. They improved my understanding of indigenous religion and the healing system. I thank all these persons with a grateful heart.

I am also grateful to the staff of the Assam State Archives, Dispur, Guwahati; National Archives of India, New Delhi; and Central Library, University of Delhi, New Delhi. Special mention must be made of Ms Nani Soli, Mrs Kime Ampi, Mrs Bomgam Bagra Kamduk, and Ms Kime Yare of Arunachal Pradesh State Archives, Itanagar, and Mr Kamalesh Kumar Pandey of State Library, Itanagar, for their special support in tracing the elusive old records. My stay in New Delhi was hosted by two families; I remember the love and affection of Professor Shyam Narayan Singh, Professor Nandini C. Singh, Babu, and Bani. My brother-in-law Mr Mizum Nyodu, Faculty of Law, University of Delhi, New Delhi, provided me with another home in the blazing heat of Delhi summer.

My dear wife Michak and son Jenyom have been a source of constant support and sweet distractions. Our babysitter Ms Jamuna has been an unacknowledged but important source of support. My

Ane Kai Orom Rilu Kadu Dabi bravely fought with illness and could not see the completion of this book. I dedicate this book to her. To them and all the members of my extended joint family and relatives, I owe a lot for their love, care, support, and respect they have for academics.

TAJEN DABI

Acknowledgements

Most of the contents of Chapter 2 of this book appeared as 'Medicine in British Frontier Policy: Disease, Epidemics, and Dispensaries in Arunachal Pradesh c. 1912–1947' in the *Indian Historical Review*, vol. 45, no. 1, 2018, pp. 124–50. The chapter is not a reproduction of the article, it has undergone some minor modifications for this book although the general layout and arguments remain the same. I am grateful to Sage to allow me to re-publish articles published in the *Indian Historical Review*.

The contents of Chapter 4 of this book appeared in different versions in various journals and conference proceedings. The chapter is not a replica of these publications; the layout and presentation are different. Following are the publications, which were single-authored by me: (1) 'Magical Hands: Rendezvous with a Buddhist Medicine Man', *Rajiv Gandhi University Research Journal*, vol. 14, no. 1–2, 2015, pp. 99–109; (2) 'Indigenous Healing Traditions of Arunachal Pradesh: An Overview', *Asian Journal of Research in Social Sciences and Humanities,* vol. 7, no. 11, November 2017, pp. 149–57; (3) 'Indigenous Healing Through A "Foreign" Mouth: A Case Study of a Nyishi Priest's Life and Practice, Arunachal Pradesh, India', *North Asian International Research Journal of Social Science & Humanities*, vol. 3, no. 11, November 2017, pp. 183–8; (4) 'A Priests' Chant: Healing Traditions amongst the Galo tribe, Arunachal Pradesh, India', *Saudi Journal of Humanities and Social Science*, vol. 2, no. 11, November 2017, pp. 1058–61; (5) 'Mixed Therapy: An Outline of Monpa Healing Traditions', *North Asian International Research Journal of Social Science & Humanities*, vol. 3, no. 12, December 2017, pp. 104–9; (6) 'Re-assessing Pre-Colonial Ethnomedicine: Monpa Chiropractic Tradition', in *Pre-Colonial History and Traditions of Arunachal Pradesh*, ed. Sudhir Kumar Singh and Ashan Riddi, Guwahati: DVS Publishers, 2017, pp. 122–33.

The plates appearing in this book have been sourced from the Directorate of Information and Public Relations, Government of Arunachal Pradesh, Naharlagun (DIPR, GoAP). The copyright of the picture rests with the DIPR, GoAP. I am grateful to the DIPR, GoAP for allowing me to use the pictures in this book.

The Indian Council of Historical Research (ICHR) provided travel grant for visiting archives during my PhD study, the gist of which appears in this book. I want to record my gratitude to the ICHR.

Introduction

Christianity is the most visible legacy of British rule in the hills of north-east India. The cultural legacy of the colonial and missionary influences dominates the contemporary debate as in the role of the church and Christian faith in the separatist movements in the North-East. Conversely, in the plains, the talk is about known references to colonial regimes: the coming of new revenue systems, plantation economy, labour exploitation, national upsurges, and lately, environment and ecology.

Historical scholarship on the hill societies of the eastern Himalayas traverses a gradient where one makes an easy downhill-slide to gather the nature of Ahom-tribal relations, British-tribal relations, constitutional and administrative growth, and others. In these studies, the British-tribal relations are seen in terms of interventions. As a result of the limited intercourse between the peoples of Arunachal Pradesh with the colonial state, as compared with other hill regions of north-east India, the possibility of the use of medicine in British frontier policy was not speculated. This book is an attempt to contribute a new domain of knowledge in the history of British interventions in the state by exploring the medical aspects of colonial interventions and their legacy.

A recent take on the history of the region by an Oxford scholar offers a refreshing reading. M.L. Bose's *History of Arunachal* was getting 40 years old and not a single scholarship had come up to review the historical focus on the region as a whole. Guyot-Rechard's *Shadow States* questions James Scott's thesis that hill societies purposefully evade states, arguing that the North-East Frontier Agency (NEFA)[1] tribes, especially the Monpas, were willing to countenance state presence in their midst. The *Shadow States* offers an explanation citing Noel Williamson's unarmed peaceful initial expedition into the Siang valley: rather than possessed of an innate drive to escape the state, NEFA's inhabitants were averse to a certain kind of state presence—a presence based primarily on the use of violent coercion or the constant possibility for it and precluding local agency.[2]

The primary motivation in the tribal-government relationship, according to Guyot-Rechard, was the 'Paradox of vulnerability ... vulnerability had defined the Indian state as it expanded in the 1950s, and people had accepted this expansion not in spite or ignorance of this vulnerability, but partly because of it'.[3] Speaking of the psychological effects of the Chinese aggression and its political fallout, she argues:

> If occupation had shown some local communities that China could deliver, and in very little time, it had also shown that they themselves had little control over what it delivered. The Indian state, by contrast, was fragile and imperfect; but its tensions, its vulnerabilities, its reliance on the population, and perhaps its focus on relief and rehabilitation offered more space to negotiate, criticize, and make demands.[4]

Since the use of medicine in the colonial frontier policy in the North East Frontier Tract (NEFT) received cursory mention in the extant historical research, the book might appear simple and uncomplicated with an overdose of data charting out the growth of medical policy and healthcare institutions. It is but in this mundane exercise that the strength of this book lies: in the presentation of a new set of data to chart a divergent course of colonial interventions in the eastern Himalayas, one dotted with the targeted use of medicine since the late colonial period (in the context of India and Assam); absence of missionary activities in 'humanizing', not to speak of education and medical mission, the tribes; and, how the postcolonial Indian state approached the people and the question of integration of the region. Just as the study of colonialism and postcolonial Indian state cannot, and should not, be restricted to a monolithic view of colonialism and the nation, the nature of relationships between governments and un-administered regions on its edge need not always be assumed to have taken a pre-identified course catalysed by known forms of contacts and negotiations. It is hoped that this book will provide, if not provoke, an extra layer of historical imagination when writing about the recent history of the frontier.

Ethnography for History and What This History is About

Writing a history on and about pre-literate societies leads one to the castle of ethnology. Edward Evans-Pritchard once pointed out that anthropologists write contemporaneous history.[5] Furer-Haimendorf instead argued that the traditions of synchronic studies established by Malinowski and Radcliffe-Brown did not favour a sustained interest in historical processes, and the timescale of the average type of fieldwork has set limits to the anthropologist's ability to observe social processes over extended periods. To erase such lacunae, Furer-Haimendorf suggested an expanded time span for anthropological fieldwork from twenty to more than thirty years to enable the evaluation of processes of change and transformation of a society experienced under the impact of the contact with materially more advanced populations or of environmental change.[6] In contrast to the British and the American anthropologists, who do research far away from their homes in a completely different cultural environment, the approach and amount of time dedicated to fieldwork for Indian anthropologists researching in India is different.[7] The analysis of aspects of traditions related to ailments and health among the communities of the region sits on the shoulders of such giants who take a positive view of *emic* perspectives. Extant literature, brief field studies, and interviews supplement the idea of ethnological knowledge this book pretends to outline. This being the sad case, it is asserted that the use, or abuse, of ethnography in this book is solely for the ends of history.

Commenting on the inclination to view Western biomedicine as another face of capitalism, Lynn M. Morgan says that medicine under capitalism is one thing, but medicine as capitalism is problematic.[8] Whether a political economy of the healthcare system in Arunachal is a viable concept before one has a healthcare history at hand cannot be argued too far. And to do the same thing concurrently is something this book does not promise. No attempt is being made at understanding the nature of colonial ethnography and its implied morality; the information found therein is treated in situ.[9] Morgan urged for a complete political economy of health approach to include historical perspective, conflict of dialectical models of social change, and a theory of disease causation that is multifactorial and encompasses social aetiology.[10] Such studies will also include anthropological concepts like historical trauma and help expand the scope of traditional epidemiological studies by drawing on factors from the past to explain the social and spatial distribution of contemporary health problems.[11] Even by way of excuse, then, it is submitted that a fertile ground for scholarship exists on themes this book takes a shallow look into: studies on food habits, indigenous midwifery, bonesetters, chiropractors, herbal experts, and ritual healers.

Further studies at the micro-level might unearth a different category of data (both archival and field-based), complement, or contest the findings and specific arguments of this book. But on the general principles and the basic arguments, the existence of colonial medical policy, the absence of medical missions, and medicine as the most important agency of state mediation, the authenticity of facts and the novelty of presentation is claimed.

Viewing the indigenous healing traditions vis-à-vis other religious healing practices only through the prism of cultural 'invasion' limits the scope of sound academic understanding of such processes; the tendency is not dissimilar in the current researches on Arunachal, especially by indigenous scholars. To suppose an indigenous-healing-system-versus-Western-medicine scenario would require at least two known determinants to have priorly taken place such that the process has churned up enough social impacts for a meaningful historical analysis—that of penetration of modern medicine extensively into the hills, and the presence of medical mission. The first factor is weak until now and the second was absent. The primary focus of the book is on the ideological and institutional aspects of the development of the modern healthcare system.

In part, this story explains why, ideologically, Arunachal is different from the other restive tribal areas of north-east India. It will inform, as a case study, the comparative analysis of government policies in contested/conflict zones. In assessing the role of medicine in expanding government influence, this book contributes existing views on the nature of contact between the British and the tribes as well as in assessing how governments appropriate regions outside regular administrative limits within the bounds of the state when military occupation is not resorted to or required. The book shifts the focus of analysing colonial and government medical policy from the 'centre' to the 'periphery', the metros to the hinterland, and from the plains to the hills. It also delineates the commonalities and contrasts in the medical policy of the two ideologically different regimes during whose brief period Arunachal emerged into the political and psychological topography of the modern state.

Understanding Colonial Medicine: A Glance

Studies abound on the themes of disease and epidemics in history as also about the rise of hospitals and the emergence of Western medicine. The colonial medical policy and medical administration in India too has already attracted remarkable scholarships to be repeated here. As this book shows subsequently, the idea of colonial medicine in its classic sense of 'colonizing the body' did not operate in Arunachal. Hence it won't be a very fruitful exercise to engage the readers' minds to the otherwise exhaustive and original works relating to colonial medicine within India and elsewhere. Wherever needed, due reference and comparisons have been made to posit the state of the medical policy of the frontier with others.

However, a short invocation to the sea gods always offers some measure of reassurance and safety when embarking on a rough voyage in a makeshift dugout. This might also be of some assistance to the general readers to know about some of the major works on the subject. Locating the role of science and technology during colonial expansion became a major area of research since the 1980s. D.R. Headrick's *The Tools of Empire: Technology and European Imperialism in the Nineteenth Century* (1981) was one of the earliest of such works. Headrick showed how the penetration of Africa would not have been possible without conquering disease. Phillip D. Curtin's *Death by Migration: Europe's Encounter with the Tropical World in the Nineteenth Century* (1989) highlights the challenges faced by the British in tropical India in terms of epidemics and diseases.

Roy MacLeod and Lewis Milton's edited work *Disease, Medicine and Empire: Perspectives of Western Medicine and the Experience of European Expansion* (1988) is a critical account of colonial medical policies in Africa, Asia, and Australia. David Arnold's edited book *Imperial Medicine and Indigenous Societies* (1988) contains essays on European medical policies in India, New Zealand (Maoris), the Belgian Congo, Philippines, and Southern Rhodesia. Insanity, smallpox, medicine and racial politics, sleeping sickness, cholera, plague, influenza, and malnutrition are the themes of focus. Charles Leslie's edited volume, *Asian Medical Systems: A Comparative Study* (1976) provides insight into the relationship between modern and traditional medicine. Leslie argues in his introduction that Asian medical systems provide fascinating opportunities both to directly observe practices that continue ancient scientific modes of thought and to analyse the historical processes that mediate their relationship to modern science and technology. The book also highlights the inadequacies of terms like 'modern medicine', 'scientific medicine', 'Western medicine', etc.[12] Taylor, while speaking in the context of Ayurveda, predicts that indigenous medical practice will slowly fade into a synthesis with scientific medicine.[13]

There are equally many authoritative works specific to India. The best known in this regard is David Arnold's *Colonizing the Body: State, Medicine and Epidemic Diseases in Nineteenth-century India* (1993). This work speaks about the mixture of dissent and desire, the hateful and the hegemonic in what is a 'paradoxical Indian response to Western medicine'.[14] The change from the Indian resistance of Western medicine to its adoption by the emerging political elite is another theme highlighted in the book. This suggests that colonial medicine, not motivated by any altruistic feelings for the Indians, was gradually accepted by the educated class. The Western healthcare system was part of the colonial reordering of Indian society and its values, and so its acceptance by the middle class reflected the changing nature of indigenous outlook on Western institutions and values.

Poonam Bala's *Imperialism and Medicine in Bengal: A Socio-Historical Perspective* (1991) as a description of the professionalization of imperial medicine throws light on medical history and its social dimension. The work analyses the interaction between practitioners of indigenous drugs and imperial policies and perspectives. Deepak Kumar's *Science and the Raj 1857–1905* (1995) explores the development of science under the colonial situation, its social implications, and its economic ramification. Kumar outlines the military roots of medical service and how medical education in

Victorian India was shaped by imperial prerogatives.[15] Anil Kumar's *Medicine and the Raj: British Medical Policy in India, 1835–1911* (1998) unravels the whole gamut of policies and ideological nuances related to medicine, outlining in one volume the growth of medical education, hospitals, pharmacies, medical service, disease, and medical research.

With a similar perspective, Biswamoy Pati and Mark Harrison's edited work *Health, Medicine and Empire: Perspectives on Colonial India* (2001) addresses specific issues of varying themes. The editors in their introduction speak about how social historians treat epidemics as windows through which to view colonial society. The publication of the proceedings of the *61st Session of the Indian History Congress, 2001* consisting of different themes on medical and social history may be considered an updated and expanded work along similar lines. Edited by Deepak Kumar and titled *Disease and Medicine in India: A Historical Overview* (2001), the volume covers a variety of essays and articles on medical traditions of pre-modern India and issues during modern India.

In all these works, not a single chapter is on Assam or north-east India. The absence is baffling given the fact that Assam formed one of the capitalist districts of the East India Company (EIC) long before many provinces of the country. And it is in the hills of north-east India that one can find the missionary works (in education as in medical works) in full gear during the colonial period. With data mined from local archives, a sub-section is presented later on the roots of the colonial medical policy in the Brahmaputra valley during the nineteenth century. This is not comprehensive but will offer a tentative account of the colonial roots of modern medicine in Assam until improvised by a specialized study on the matter.

Before that, a few lines on some works that border on ethnohistory. An edited volume by Chittabrata Palit and Achintya Dutta entitled *History of Medicine in India: The Medical Encounter* (2011) deals with the medical encounter between Eastern and Western medicine. The work is an attempt to counter the 'Western views' of historians like Phillip Curtin, David Arnold, Ralph Nicholas, Roy McLeod, Mark Harrison, and others. Western medicine extensively borrowed indigenous medical knowledge and its dominance of Western medicine was enshrined through the institutions of the colonial state.[16] While critiquing the British medical policy in India, the authors make a significant remark: 'India was not the *White-man's grave*; rather she became the graveyard of Indians under British rule'.[17]

Lancy Lobo's recently published book *Malaria in the Social Context: A Study of Western India* (2010) examines traditional knowledge systems in conjunction with biomedical elements to promote effective health education in western India. Babul Roy's work *Medical Anthropology: Studies in the Highlands of Assam* (2012) studies the cultural determinants of disease, sickness, and illness amongst the Dimasa Kachari and Zeme Naga of Assam. Roy also studies the traditional pharmacopoeia and the role and function of traditional medical practitioners.

Coolies, Cholera, and Tea Gardens: Colonial Medical Policy in the Brahmaputra Valley

It appears that no sooner had the British wrested Assam from the Burmese, their attention was drawn more to diseases and native habits than to consolidate their position. This is what some of the earliest European memoirs suggest: the confrontation of diseases in Cachar;[18] Assam as a place where a human footstep was unknown and the atmosphere, even to the natives themselves, pregnant with febrile miasma and death;[19] the 'natural obstacles' and opium-eating habit of the natives was responsible for the spread of cholera;[20] opium as one of the greatest obstacles to the advancement and prosperity of Assam;[21] the disposal of the dead; [22] and, the general sultry environment. The projected unhealthy environment of

Assam and lack of sanitation fuelled the miasmatic theory of disease.

It was against this backdrop that epidemics were reported. In May–June 1834, an epidemic of cholera spread to Dhaka, Jumalpur, Goalpara, Guwahati, and Bishwanath which reportedly took away a large portion of the population of Assam.[23] Informed by miasmatic theory, sanitation and environment began to guide the choice of location of military stations. For example, the 'Sudder Station' of north-central Assam was shifted from Darrang to Tezpur in 1835 to escape the disease.[24] Once settled at the desired station, hospitals and dispensaries were established. As elsewhere in India, the position of the doctors in the Brahmaputra valley was not given importance in the official hierarchy. A description of a hospital at Guwahati throws light on this aspect:

> Only one Assistant Surgeon, with the help of an Apothecary, and four or five Native Doctors, is allowed for the double duties of Gohatti. The Civil charge is of itself unusually heavy, yet he is called upon to perform the duties of the Sebundy Corps besides. ... The Medical Officer at Gohatti has always been placed in an anomalous footing as to pay and allowances ... In no part of India is the inferiority of pay of the Medical Officer so much felt as in Assam.[25]

The establishment of hospitals and the gradual development of colonial medical policy in the Brahmaputra valley was intimately linked to the tea industry. Soon after the signing of the Treaty of Yandaboo (1826) tea gardens were started in Assam. The first such garden was opened in Sadiya in 1826 by the brother of Lt. Bruce of the Royal Navy who oversaw patrolling of the river Kundil.[26] The British found that the native Assamese were unwilling to work in the labour-intensive industry[27] and forced conscription in a newly acquired province was not a wise alternative. The indentured labours from central India provided the easy solution.

The colonial authorities brought labourers by steamer via the ports of Bengal to Assam; waterways being the (only) viable means of communication then. Disease and epidemics brought in by these migrant workers provided the first impetus towards the evolution of a colonial medical policy in Assam. On 1 June 1861 Lieutenant Colonel H. Vitch, the Officiating Judicial Commissioner of Assam wrote to Henry Hopkinson, Commissioner of Assam:

So very frequent re-appearance of Cholera in Assam in late years, has been disseminated by these importations of coolies infested with that disease ... sanitary measures should be adopted to prevent the importation of coolies infested by this, or any other dangerous disease, not only in justice to the crews and passengers of these steam vessels, but as a protection to Assam against a disease which is carrying off the population by thousands as compared with the few hundreds of imported labourers brought to the country ... to effect same system of inspection and sanitary requirements for coolies embarked to Assam as those shipped to colonies...[28]

Hopkinson, in turn, wrote to the Secretary to the Government of Bengal and relayed the threat of disease brought by the coolies in Assam and urged for suitable steps to be taken immediately to control the menace. The result came in the form of a prescriptive order:

With a view to prevent the spread of Cholera in the interior of tea districts by gangs of labourer imported ... it is hereby notified ... that whenever Cholera has appeared on board any vessel, or fleet of boats conveying labourers to the tea districts, whether in charge of gardens sirdars or not, the labourers destined for any place of debarkation instead of being landed at that place, when the steamer or boats arrive there, shall be landed under the orders of the Magistrate at some selected place at a reasonable distance from the station, and kept under observation for such time as the medical officer in charge of the station or debarkation depot may consider advisable. In furtherance of this object Cholera camps have been established at Seebsagar, Gowhatty, and Durrung in the Assam...[29]

The order was not without reason: in 1873, the outbreak of cholera and the resultant death of four workers out of 160 aboard a steamer named 'Panjab' docking at Goalpara created panic in the administration.[30] The epidemic generated interest in epidemiology so that fruitful measures could be undertaken.[31] A Sanitary Commissioner for Assam was appointed in 1868.[32] 'Cholera camps' for observation of the newly imported workers were established at Sibsagar, Guwahati, and Dibrugarh.[33] 'Charitable Dispensaries' were started at Barpeta, Guwahati, Tezpur, Naogaon, Sibsagar, Dibrugarh, North Lakhimpur, Samagoodting, and Shillong.[34]

It was only after the immediate medical needs of the tea gardens and European Officers were met that medical facilities were gradually extended to the civilians.[35] The Charitable Dispensaries were even not funded by the government at this period and only the pay of the serving doctors was partially met by the state. The position of the dispensaries was similar to what was prevalent in other parts of India:

> The support originally given by the Government to Charitable Dispensaries consisted of a monthly payment equal to the amount realised from local subscriptions. In the year 1854 this system was changed. Money payment was done away with; but whenever the residents of a station made over a building for an Hospital or Dispensary, and guaranteed an average monthly income, Government undertook to appoint a Sub-Assistant Surgeon or a Native Doctor, according as the monthly sum subscribed should equal the pay of one or the other of those grades. The salary of the Medical Officer, with free medicines from the Government stores, was thus to represent the measure of Government support; and no pecuniary allowance of any kind or on any account was to be given. All applications made to the Government since 1864, on behalf of Charitable Dispensaries, have been dealt with in the spirit of these orders.[36]

The expansion of the medical department followed the administrative expansion after Assam was separated from Bengal. In the year 1903, the Medical Department in Assam was divided into two branches: the Inspector-General of Civil Hospitals (IGCH) headed the department while the Sanitary Commissioner dealt with all questions of purely sanitary character.[37] The process of expansion of hospitals and health centres were determined not by population but by strategic and economic importance. This is evident from a comparison of the population of some important towns and the types of hospitals opened there as given in Appendix IX.

In Assam, conflicts between indigenous beliefs and colonial medicine were reported. Smallpox was identified with the Goddess Sitala, whose awesome presence was manifested through the disease. Deliverance from possession by the goddess was sought through songs, prayers, devotional offerings, and cooling potions.[38] Local medics sought cure through the process of variolation, a practice banned by the Vaccination Act of the 1870s and 1880s.[39] And since vaccination defiled the goddess, popular distrust against it spread; some see this as an important site of cultural resistance to colonial medical intervention in Assam.[40]

Notes

1. The North-East Frontier Agency (hereafter NEFA) was the former administrative and academically well-known name of Arunachal Pradesh. Till the 1950s, the term was synonymously used with the North-East Frontier Tract (hereafter NEFT). Please see Table 1.1 for a glance of the administrative growth of the state. For the sake of brevity, I have used 'Arunachal' in this book, except in the tables and notes, instead of using the longish 'Arunachal Pradesh'. The terms NEFT and NEFA, however, are used at appropriate places to maintain the historical context.
2. Berenice Guyot-Rechard, *Shadow States: India, China and the Himalayas, 1910–1962*, Cambridge: Cambridge University Press, 2017, p. 119.

3. Ibid., pp. 128, 249.
4. Ibid., p. 250.
5. As quoted in Christoph von Furer-Haimendorf, 'The Presidential Address-1976', *RAIN*, vol. na, no. 18, February 1977, pp. 6–11.
6. Furer-Haimendorf, 'The Presidential Address', p. 6. Furer-Haimendorf followed his dictum and came to do research on the Apatanis in the early 1980s, four decades after he first worked amongst them.
7. Andre Beteille in the 'Introduction' to Nirmal Kumar Bose, *The Structure of Hindu Society*, tr. Andre Beteille, 3rd revd edn, Hyderabad: Orient Longman, 1994, pp. 12–13.
8. Lynn M. Morgan, 'Dependency Theory in the Political Economy of Health: An Anthropological Critique', *Medical Anthropology Quarterly,* New Series 1, no. 2, June 1987, pp. 131–54, 138.
9. Among others, expositions on such themes can be found in Meena Radhakrishnan, 'Of Apes and Ancestors: Evolutionary Science and Colonial Ethnography', *The Indian Historical Review*, vol. XXXIII, no. 1, Jan. 2006, pp. 1–23; and David Hardiman, 'Knowledge System of the Bhils', *The Indian Historical Review*, vol. xxxiii, no. 1, Jan. 2006, pp. 202–24.
10. Morgan, 'Dependency Theory', p. 132.
11. Barbara D. Miller, *Cultural Anthropology*, 7th edn, New York: Pearson Education, 2012, p. 177.
12. Charles Leslie, ed., *Asian Medical Systems: A Comparative Study*, London: University of California Press, 1976, pp. 6–7.
13. Carl E. Taylor, 'The Place of Indigenous Medical Practitioners in the Modernization of Health Services', as cited in Leslie, ed., *Asian Medical Systems*, p. 298.
14. As reflected in Biswamoy Pati and Mark Harrison, eds., *Health, Medicine and Empire Perspectives on Colonial on Colonial*, New Delhi: Orient Longman, 2001, p. 19.
15. Deepak Kumar, *Science and the Raj, 1857–1905*, Delhi: Oxford University Press, 1995, p. 109.
16. Chittabrata Palit and Achintya Dutta, eds., *History of Medicine in India: The Medical Encounter*, Delhi: Kalpaz Publications, 2011, p. 15.
17. Palit and Dutta, *History of Medicine*, p. 17.

18. Robert Boileau Pemberton, *The Eastern Frontier of India*, 1835; repr., New Delhi: Mittal Publications, 2015, pp. 208–9.
19. John M' Cosh, *Topography of Assam*, New Delhi, Logos Press, 2000, p. 13.
20. W.W. Hunter, *Statistical Account of Assam*, vol. I, London: Trübner & Co., 1879, p. 96.
21. 'Memorandum by Mr. W.G. Young on certain matters to which his attention was attracted during his recent trips to Assam,' Government of Bengal, File No. 277/604 of 1857–58, pp. 1–8, paragraph no. 13, Assam State Archives (hereafter ASA), Dispur.
22. M' Cosh, *Topography*, pp. 111–13.
23. Ibid., p. 114.
24. Ibid., p. 93.
25. Ibid., pp. 91–2.
26. L.W. Shakespear, *History of the Assam Rifles*, 1929; repr., Sussex, England: Naval and Military Press, 2005, p. 40.
27. 'Memorandum by Mr. W.G. Young on certain matters to which his attention was attracted during his recent trips to Assam,' Government of Bengal, File No. 277/604 of 1857–58, pp. 1–8, paragraph no. 13, ASA, Dispur.
28. File No. 375 of 1861, Government of Bengal, ASA, Dispur.
29. File No. 139/249 of 1869–72, Government of Bengal, ASA, Dispur.
30. CMO to Comber, File No. 49/87 of 1873, Government of Bengal Papers-5, ASA, Dispur.
31. Nicholson to Grant, File No. 49/87 of 1873, Government of Bengal Papers-5, ASA, Dispur.
32. Baylay to the Commissioner of Assam, Government of Bengal Paper, Nos. 1–2, File No. 649 of 1868, ASA, Dispur.
33. File No. 139/249 of 1869–72, Government of Bengal, ASA, Dispur; and File No. 136/246 of 1872, Government of Bengal Papers-2, ASA, Dispur.
34. File No. 56 of 1872–74, Assam Secretariat, Nos. 1–36, ASA, Dispur.
35. Bernard to Hopkinson, File No. 138/248 of 1872, Government of Bengal Papers-4, ASA, Dispur.
36. Geoghegan to Commissioner of Assam, Letter No. 904, File No. 494 of 1864, Government of Bengal, Nos. 1–7, ASA, Dispur.

37. B.C. Allen et al., *Gazetteer of Bengal and North-East India*, 1905; rpt, New Delhi: Mittal Publication, 2012, p. 12.
38. Nirmalaprabha Bordoloi, *Assamar Loka Samskriti* as quoted in Tahir Hussain Ansari, 'Disease and Medicine in the Colonial Assam during 19th Century', *Journal of Business Management & Social Sciences Research*, vol. 2, no. 1, January 2013, p. 93.
39. Ansari, 'Disease and Medicine', p. 93.
40. Ibid.

1

Beyond the Colony

Conceiving the NEFT

Mapping resources and peoples is an enterprise that evolved as part of state regimes. From early Greek geographers to contemporary census enumerators, both the spatial and human dimensions of the surrounding environment have constantly been attempted to be calculated and categorized. The references to the geography and people of the eastern Himalayas that separates the Tibetan plateau from the Brahmaputra valley have thus started to trickle in from classical Greek sources. This continued when the region and its peoples started to be mentioned in the redacted Hindu religious texts that were produced after the establishment of Hindu state systems in the Brahmaputra valley from around the fifth century AD.

People and the Physical Environment

Being located outside the successive state systems of the Brahmaputra valley, the geography and the peoples of the region did not naturally feature much in the popular media of the times, such as in inscriptions, coins, paintings, religious texts, travelogues, official correspondences, and the like. This was so until the period of the Ahoms, the best known and the longest-reigning dynasty of Assam of Burmese origin, who ruled much of the Brahmaputra valley until the East India Company, well-footed in neighbouring Bengal, came into the picture during the closing decades of the eighteenth century.

The increase in the frequency and depth of references to the peoples of the eastern Himalayas during the Ahom times could be because of another important reason. The people themselves were late migrants to the region, at least a substantial majority of them. This is what numerous myth and migration theories have presently revealed.[1] Most communities of the region migrated from Tibet and the east, in batches, probably over centuries starting roughly from the fifth century. The Akas (Hrusso) of Kameng traces their origin from a mythical king of the plains. The Buddhist communities (excepting the Khamptis and Singphos), who dwell in the present Tibetan-Indian borderland and who paid taxes to Tibetan officials till the 1950s, were the southern extensions of the monastic Tibetan state.

This suggests a slow and sparse peopling of the region.[2] The northern bank of the Brahmaputra valley itself was a very thinly populated region till the colonial period.[3] No statistics or data about the demography of the region is available until the 1961 census, but it is not unwise to presume that population growth sufficient enough to attract the attention of the neighbouring states of the plains coincided with the Ahom period. Thus the increased references as mentioned earlier. After the East India Company (EIC) took over the reign of Assam from the second quarter of the nineteenth century, the era of more information and knowledge about both the physical geography and peoples of the region began.

The socio-political evolution in the hills of Arunachal during this period remained confined to networks of kinship ties across various groups with elements of chieftainship in some areas.[4] Geographical barriers kept people away from each other[5] and therefore social and political evolution on a composite scale did not take place.

The traditional livelihood subsistence activities depended on hunting, shifting as well as terrace agriculture, animal husbandry, barter trade, etc. Trade relations extended to Tibet in the north and

Assam in the south through numerous trade routes.[6] A kind of slave trade was another source of sustenance livelihood activities.[7] Slaves were also often brought from the plains which led to conflicts with the respective governments of the Ahom and the British. Social divisions existed in some form, defying uniform patterns across the communities. Because such divisions were not institutionalized, except in few cases, the traditional society of Arunachal has generally been described in egalitarian terms. Religious beliefs deeply influenced the worldview of the people. Religious belief often determined the lifestyle and idea of life, so it gradually became a part of customs and practices in the form of ritual, healing, omen, oath, and ordeals.[8] Even for construction of a house, rituals were offered; a similar exercise was done for hunting and almost all other important works.

Verrier Elwin had classified the communities of Arunachal into three broad artistic and cultural 'provinces'.[9] The first is, to conveniently paraphrase, the Buddhist groups: the Monpa, the Sherdukpen, the Memba, and the Khamba who live in the north near Tibet from Mechuka through Tuting, Mankhota, and Gelling to Wallong in the Lohit. Despite artistic and geographical barriers, Elwin also puts the Khampti and the Singpho, who follow Hinayana Buddhism, in this group on the basis of religion. The second group extends rather in a convenient west–east or east–west direction, from Seppa in Kameng in the west through Subansiri, Siang, and Lohit in the east on the basis of traditions of weaving, absence of woodcarving, and stress on fine work in cane and bamboo. Finally, the Noctes, many of whom are Vaishnavites by faith, along with the Wanchos and the Tangsas form the third group on the basis of Burmese influence. Thirty-five years after Elwin's classification, the Anthropological Survey of India (AnSI) offered two sets of cultural zones: the hills and the plains on the basis of geography and five zones on the basis of concentration of tribal groups.[10]

The indigenous languages spoken in the region belong to the Tibeto-Chinese family under which the Khampti-Shan belongs to the Siamese-Chinese sub-family and the rest belong to the Tibeto-Burman sub-family, making a total of more than forty-two languages.[11] According to the Census 2011, the population of the state was 13.84 lakh of which 22.94 per cent live in urban areas. Christianity is the most widely professed religion (30.24 per cent) followed by Hinduism (29.04 per cent), indigenous religion (26.24 per cent), Buddhism (11.77 per cent), Islam (1.95 per cent), Sikhism (0.24 per cent), and Jainism (0.06 per cent).[12]

Located in the extreme north-eastern corner of India, Arunachal shares an international boundary with Bhutan in the west, China in the north, and Myanmar in the east. It also shares its boundary with the state of Assam in the south and Nagaland in the south-east. Arunachal is a land of climatic extremities and cultural diversity. It is the largest state in north-east India with the least density of population. Elevations range from 50 MSL in the foothills to about 7,000 MSL in the high snow-clad mountains, and rainfall varies from 1,000 mm. in the higher reaches to 5,750 mm. in the foothills.[13] The hills overlooking the Brahmaputra valley gradually taper off to the plains of the Brahmaputra. Much of the plains portion of the erstwhile North-East Frontier Agency (NEFA) was transferred to Assam in 1951. The mountain ranges run in a north–south direction, restricting movement within the region, but at the same time facilitating passages from north to south. Such numerous passes were the routes of traditional commerce which were linked to the *duar*s (passes in the plains where routes and trade from the hills merged) and fairs in the foothills.

The northern areas of higher altitudes with alpine vegetation experience extreme cold while the rest of the state is a mix of mountainous wet temperate and tropical evergreen vegetation with extreme climatic conditions. Five big rivers along with their tributaries namely the Kameng, the Subansiri, the Siang, the Dibang, and the Lohit drain the state and flow into the Brahmaputra. The richness of life forms, i.e. the flora and fauna present rich biodiversity with over 5,000 species of plants, about 85 terrestrial mammals, over 500 birds, and a large number of butterflies, insects, and reptiles.[14] Such an unparalleled occurrence of life form is because of the peculiar location of the state which is at the junction of the Palaearctic, Indo-Chinese, and Indo-Malayan bio-geographic regions.[15] The rich biodiversity of the state is matched by linguistic and cultural diversity as well.

From Ethnography to the Dawn of 'History'

Writings on the peoples of the region fall within the categories of ethnology (mostly commissioned by the colonial state, as Dalton's *Descriptive Ethnology*), ethnography (specific works on particular tribes, many of which came out in the *Memoirs of the Asiatic Society*), official administrative-history (as that of Pemberton, *The Eastern Frontier of India*; Mackenzie, *The North East Frontier of India*; and Reid, *History of Frontier Areas*) during the period prior to the 1950s. Thereafter, government-sponsored anthropological works started by Christoph von Furer-Haimendorf and modelled by Verrier Elwin took a renewed interest during the 'anthropological turn' since the mid-1950s. This laid the foundation of ethnohistorical research which is now the primary occupation of contemporary local researchers, including the one saying so. Lately, even historical novels have made a welcome appearance.[16] This helped the study of the indigenous societies to 'move both forward and backward in time'.[17] A more convenient marriage between anthropology and history could not have happened.

The volumes of ethnological and historical accounts written by the European officer-travellers to professional anthropologists like Furer-Haimendorf, Verrier Elwin, and after, from the third decade of the nineteenth to the close of the twentieth century, form the pivot from where one might take a chosen trajectory of analysis and interpretation about the region and its peoples. Then, to clarify as to when and where the imprints of ethnology and history begin to influence each other and how this contributes to a broader understanding of the region begets some elaboration. After all, it is from the intersection of ethnology and history that a fuller account of the region and its peoples emerge.

It is difficult to place the histories of the various ethnic groups or the region itself under the usual categories of periodization, pre-colonial, colonial, and post-colonial.[18] But it is helpful to employ these labels and yardsticks of historical enquiry in making sense of a region where both ethnology and history have equal stake and models and analyses to offer. Chronologically, it is not difficult to establish the time when the circumstances of history brought ethnography to map the region and its peoples. From the stray and confusing references of the classical Greek accounts and the Hindu religious texts to the colonial and postcolonial accounts, the interest, intensity, and scope of ethnography sharpened and widened as the region began to be seen from the perch of state-policy (both domestic and external) of the respective powers of the Brahmaputra valley. In this sense, it was history that brought ethnography to throw light on a region peopled by pre-literate societies.

Thus, the new attention that the region attracted during the colonial period inadvertently pushed it within the rim of history. In the scheme of the expanding commercial interest of the EIC, and later the British Empire, a region that not only separated the Assam plains from Tibet but also lay on the key trade route to both China and Burma, acquired a new meaning. The imperial commercial and strategic considerations only accentuated this process. As is the contemporary reality, the region's publicity as well as importance derived much, first, from the Chinese question from the beginning of the twentieth century, and later (as now), its claim on the region. It might therefore be surmised that the push of history required ethnographic explorations of the region and its peoples to meet the ends of history itself. In the process, the 'terra incognita' and the pre-literate societies found themselves knocking at the door of 'history', asking for one to be crafted for them. How this history would be written is a debate about which scholars do not have conclusive and agreed opinion about the frame of analysis.

The publication of Scott's anarchist thesis,[19] probably the best known of the hill–plain/hill–valley binary frame of analysis, has ignited fresh interpretations about the idea of the region and its peoples. Within India, most studies choose a region-specific analysis instead of blanket generalization.[20] One such study about the eastern Himalayas argues that the region lies 'at the crossroads of the flow of ideas and commodities of states like Tibet and Assam. Yet the trajectory of its culture developed unique features in an ecological niche negotiating and interacting with other cultures' and thus emerged as a distinct region.[21]

The debate about the hill–plain divide in north-east India emerged not from the academia but ideological grumblings and politics. Soon after the independence of the country, the hills of the north-east flared up in secessionist movements, first started by the Nagas and later followed by the Mizos. The ideological roots of these separatist movements were traced to the colonial policy of segregation of the hills from the plains. Western (English) education, Christianity, and adoption of Western ways of life, it was believed, actively fomented and fertilized the seeds of separatism. This is an issue too known to be elaborated on and digressed from the primary focus of this book.

This brings us to consider the question of how the eastern Himalayas stand in the above debate. This requires a bit of elaboration. Within the 'reach' of history, the region experienced two different states, the Ahom and the British colonial states, exercising influences with varying degrees but never directly administered by either.[22] The Ahom rulers negotiated peace with various groups to discourage raids on their territory. The inchoate relations between the Ahom state and the peoples are reflected by the use of negative adjectives to refer to the latter. This trend continued during the colonial period.

Initially, the colonial authorities did not bring many alterations in the frontier policy they inherited from the Ahoms. But unlike the Ahoms, the commercial and strategic considerations required the colonial state to explore and redefine how it related itself to the peoples and the region. This led to the formulation of new policies on *posa*,[23] the introduction of the Inner Line,[24] and the generation of topographical and ethnographic details of the region and the peoples. Compared to the Ahoms, ironically, it was during the colonial period that both the segregation and the engagement with the frontier tribes of the eastern Himalayas began in a more consequential way. However, two things might be kept in mind: first, the segregation executed through the Inner Line Regulation 1873 generally blocked avenues for deeper hills–plains 'symbiotic' relationships to take root; and second, the growing engagement with the peoples happened between the tribes and the colonial state only (not the plains as a whole), at the pace and site determined by the colonial state. This book deals with one such important site. The administrative mechanisms as evolved by the colonial state and afterwards, which provided the 'constitutional frame' to the region, is given in Table 1.1.

Table 1.1 Administrative Growth of Arunachal Pradesh

Year	*Notes*
Up to 1912	'Administered' by APO Sadiya, subordinate to the Deputy Commissioner, Lakhimpur under the Dibrugarh Frontier Tract (DFT)
1912	DFT ceased to exist; Sadiya Frontier Tract District formed as a separate entity under a Political Officer and three APOs, reporting directly to the Chief Commissioner; Headquarters at Sadiya
1914	Central and Eastern Section; Headquarters at Sadiya with a Political Officer Western Section, Headquarters at Charduar with a Political Officer

contd.

Year	*Notes*	
1919	Central and Eastern Section renamed as Sadiya Frontier Tract; Western Section renamed as Balipara Frontier Tract	
1937	Start of 'actual administration'; Governor of Assam takes over the independent administration of the North-East Frontier, assisted by a Secretary; 'Governor's Secretariat' established.	
1943	Attempt to bring under normal administration, a policy of 'gradual penetration' adopted. Adviser to the Governor of Assam created by the Government of India especially for the North-East Frontier.	
1943	Tirap Frontier Tract comes into being by bifurcating certain areas from the Lakhimpur and Sadiya Frontier Tract	
1946	Balipara Frontier Tract is divided into (a) Sela Sub-Agency; and (b) the Subansiri Area	
1948	Sadiya Frontier Tract is divided into (a) Abor Hills District; and (b) Mishmi Hills District	
1951	Plains portions transferred to Assam.	
1954	The NEFT was renamed as the North-East Frontier Agency (NEFA) under NEF Area (Administration) Regulation, 1954 Reconstitution of administrative units:	
	Old Names	New Names
	Balipara Frontier Tract:	(a) Kameng Frontier Division (b) Subansiri Frontier Division
	Tirap Frontier Tract	Tirap Frontier Division
	Abor Hills District	Siang Frontier Division
	Mishmi Hills District	Lohit Frontier Division
	Naga Tribal Area	Tuensang Frontier Division
1957	Tuensang Frontier Division merged with the newly constituted Naga Hills Tuensang Area	
1965	The remaining 5 frontier divisions were renamed as follows:	
	Old Name	New Name
	Kameng Frontier Division	Kameng District
	Subansiri Frontier Division	Subansiri District
	Tirap Frontier Division	Tirap District
	Siang Frontier Division	Siang District
	Lohit Frontier Division	Lohit District

contd.

Year	*Notes*
1972	NEFA upgraded to Union Territory and renamed as Arunachal Pradesh
1987	Statehood

Sources: Reid, *History of Frontier Areas*, Chaps. 4 and 5; and Luthra, *Constitutional and Administrative Growth*, pp. 9–16.

Situating the Region within the Empire and the Nation

Recent work on the British Empire classifies the constituents of the British 'world system' into the following: colonies of rule; settlement colonies; protectorates; condominiums; mandates; naval and military fortresses; 'occupations'; treaty ports and 'concessions'; 'informal' colonies; and, 'spheres of interference'.[25] The NEFT was located right before one of the strategic 'spheres of interference'—Tibet, and on the edge[26] of Assam valley-based 'colony of rule'. It was not until the 1940s that concrete measures were taken to devise some sort of proper administrative control over parts of the region.

Starting from the establishment of the Sadiya outpost (after the First Anglo-Burmese War, 1824–6) right to World War II, the region remained a frontier juggled between numerous regulations and acts in tune with the changing colonial frontier policy but never administered. The Inner Line, an elastic and improperly defined line so named after the Inner Line Regulation of 1873 (it was officially called a 'Regulation for the Peace and Good Governance of Certain Districts of the Eastern Frontier') devised to protect the tea gardens from tribal raids, effectively kept the NEFT beyond administrative limits. In the wake of World War II, the government pushed for extending what was termed 'Control Areas' into the hills of the region. On 21 May 1941, the Government of India extended the 'Control Area' in the Sadiya Frontier Tract in Siang valley up to the McMahon Line.[27] The promulgation of the Assam Frontier (Administration of Justice) Regulation,

1945, meant to 'consolidate and amend the law governing the administration of justice in Balipara, Lakhimpur, Sadiya and Tirap Frontier Tracts of Assam'[28] reflected the move to gradually bring the frontier tract under a regular administrative mechanism.

Many studies on the nature of British tribal relations in the region tend to be shaped by the subsequent reality, i.e. the NEFT as an integral part of India, administratively. This was, however, not the case. The region which lay outside the cultural and state systems of the Brahmaputra valley until the mid-twentieth century is a product of the imperial strategic legacy rather than a regular remnant of the colony and its market. To visualize a scenario where it stands amongst the annexed hill territories of north-east India, and therefore having the same degree of forms of colonial exploitation or influence as in rebellions or Christianization is akin to picking an elephant out of a cage. As elaborated in the first part of the Introduction to this book, the region was at best provided with touring window administrators, who, as representatives of the itinerant governance,[29] were tasked to ensure peace along the Inner Line and to keep a vigil on the Tibetan border.

While World War II necessitated a separate 'adviser' for the Governor of Assam for the region, the post-independent Indian state was happy to keep the affairs of the region in the roster of the Ministry of External Affairs until the Chinese gave a gentle but firm knock in the autumn of 1962. To approach the history of the region without these important footnotes and peculiarities, as this study on medical policy and healthcare tries to show, is bound to limit the levels of entry and layers of interpretation.

Ignoring this administrative reality creates space for sweeping ex post facto criminalization of the colonial policies in order to generate a 'patriotic' past of the frontier. No less than a prominent historian of the region once lamented:

> There is a tendency even at highly responsible quarters to condemn the British or their agents [for] whatever they did in India. … It would be

highly ungenerous ... an act of ingratitude to start a campaign of vilification against that very agency which rendered yeoman service in regenerating the Assamese at a crucial period apart from redeeming the primitive tribes from their utter backwardness.[30]

More recent work extends this logic with respect to the history of the church: 'Both the hagiographies of the insider chroniclers and the stern critiques of the missionary as colonialism's Trojan horse have together had a marked tendency to undervalue an appreciation of intercultural exchanges'.[31] As a result, retrospective views on the British frontier policy in the region have often been coloured by an uncomplicated yet appealing 'colonial exploitation–tribal response' scheme.

The ideological background and instances of such vapid, linear exploration of the British-tribes relationship are not difficult to unravel. Instances of how the political issues were discussed in historical disguise are not new.[32] The debate over the assimilation-isolation approach to the tribal policy dominated the early decades of Independence, both in policy circles and academia.[33] In the case of Arunachal, a middle ground was successfully proposed by Nehru's 'missionary' Verrier Elwin—'make haste slowly'.[34] Positive as well as a critical assessment of the Nehru-Elwin policy continues to clog the pages of many contemporary writings on the region. One of them blames Elwin for the latter's 'inability to alter the colonial tribal policies such as the Inner Line Regulations'.[35] On the contrary, another recent view credits the policy as 'remarkable in weaving into bureaucratic planning a cosmogenetic mission ... to create a "local-national continuum" for cultural conservation and creativity'.[36] The eruption of an ideological divide over patronage to the tribes of the region had also spread in medical policy, a theme subsequently, and for the first time, taken up in this book.

There was another dimension to the assimilation-isolation debate. This presently appears to have been forgotten, or rather taken over, by the more dominant and appealing strait-jacket hill–plain divide analogy, both on the assumptions about how the respective societies differed and how concerned intellectuals and historians viewed it.

The position of the Assamese intelligentsia on the issue deserves belated attention in this regard. In the realm of policy decisions regarding the tribes of Arunachal (as well as other hill areas of the North-East), the Assamese intellectuals and leaders have always had a, viewed from the vantage of their own experience and (unfulfilled) aspirations, justifiable grudge, first against the British and later against the then NEFA administration (and by their own open admission, the Government of India, perceived to be represented by the Hindi lobby).

Soon after Nehru put Verrier Elwin in charge of formulating and guiding the policy of Panchsheel to enable the people of NEFA 'to develop in the lines of their own genius',[37] the Assam Sahitya Sabha, the premier and influential literary-cum-intellectual body of Assam, welcomed the delegates of the 63rd Session of the Indian National Congress with a vituperative compendium on the 'systemic propaganda from interested quarters in the rest of India against the Assamese people in relation to our Hill brethren'.[38] With spirited essays by many leading Assamese intellectuals of the day, the monograph's emphasis was twofold: to buttress the 'age-old' amity between Assam and the hill 'brethren' of Arunachal, and to expose the deliberate policy of separating the hill peoples from Assam through constitutional, administrative, and linguistic policy. The Assamese fear was not unfounded. In the wake of Chinese aggression, a separate political entity for NEFA was being visualized, and for that to happen, a cultural barrier was equally necessary to complete the process.[39]

Some important inferences may be drawn from the Assamese swansong against what they correctly realized as their gradual and unstoppable loss of the erstwhile hill districts and tracts once administered from Assam. Of these, Arunachal (along with Nagaland), where a pidgin of Assamese, Nefamese (like the Nagamese) had emerged as a lingua franca, was seen as a natural extension of the Catholic Assamese culture. The Assamese resented the post-independent central government, not least the NEFA Administration under Elwin's influence, as much as they differed with and hated the British in so far as the affairs of NEFA was concerned. This provides a division within the 'plains' section of the hill–plain ideological divide over the future of the region. While, as Indians, the Assamese intellectuals shared the same boat in their criticism of the British policy vis-à-vis isolation of the tribes, they nonetheless found their idea of greater Assam dissected by the ulterior motives from Delhi soon after the white chaps packed their bags and took the flight to London.

At the time of the annexation of north-east India by the British, there were six major tribal states under the Hinduized rulers—the Koch, the Tripuri, the Jayantiya, the Kachari, the Ahom, and the Meitei states.[40] Speaking of the present states of the region except for Arunachal, the others are successors of either (a) a preceding state system/chiefdoms; or (b) the erstwhile Christianized hill districts. Nagaland, Meghalaya, and Mizoram belong to the latter category while Tripura, Manipur, and Assam themselves belong to the former classification. In some areas, both (a) and (b) overlap as in the case of Meghalaya. This scenario suggests that region formation in north-east India in the era of nation-state, in its territorial and jurisdictional sense, had been shaped by conditions that developed during the pre-colonial and colonial period.

Arunachal stands as an example of a different yet interesting order of political evolution amongst the entire tribal areas of India. While the tribes of 'mainland' India attracts the attention of anthropologists to study the 'tribe-caste continuum', that of the hills of the North-East is the site to study the (ill-) effects of colonial policy and Christianization on the process of nation-making. Arunachal is an ideal case of how a region outside the cultural and social matrix of the Indic civilization, as well as beyond the influence of the missionaries and direct colonial administration, can be successfully nurtured into the emerging space and imagination of the culturally diverse Indian nation-state.

The credit for the exclusive identity of Arunachal must go to the colonial policy of segregation. In times of historical novels, it is not very fanciful to imagine that were it not for such policies, the region might have well become feudatories to the Burmese or the tax-extracting monastic Tibetan state. Just as one by-product of colonization was the political and administrative unification of India, one important result of the colonial commercial and strategic concern in the North-East was the demarcation, though still contested, of the border between Tibet and India.[41] The nucleus of the hill–plain divide, as rightly accused by many, was started by the British, administratively, and which later on acquired constitutional garbs, first through the Government of India Act 1935 ('Excluded Tracts') and then by the gradual emergence of the NEFA as a Union Territory.

Notes

1. Nearly every ethnographic and historical work on the tribes of the region makes a study of the myth and migration theories; M.L. Bose, *History of Arunachal Pradesh,* New Delhi: Concept Publishing, 1977, pp. 16–21, provides a revised and short account on it. A recent view on it is to be found in Stuart Blackburn, 'Memories of Migration: Notes on Legends and Beads in Arunachal Pradesh, India', *European Bulletin of Himalayan Research*, vols. 25/26, no. na, 2003/2004, pp. 16–60.
2. For an exposition on the topic see B.M. Das, *The Peoples of Assam*, Delhi: Gian Publishing House, 1987, pp. 16–63; and B.S. Mipun and Debendrak Nayak, 'A Geographical Background to Peopling of North-East India: A Study in the Dynamics of Identity and Inter-group Relations', in *Dynamics of Identity and Inter-group Relations*, ed. Kailash S. Aggarwal, Shimla: Indian Institute of Advanced Studies, 1999, pp. 17–28.
3. The whole of present Bhutan, Arunachal Pradesh, both the Assam valleys, parts of Bengal, and even parts of Orissa have been estimated as the

extent of the Pragjyotisha-Kamarupa kingdom according to both the contemporary texts and historical studies. See Nirode Boruah, *Historical Geography of Early Assam*, Guwahati: DVS Publisher, 2010, pp. 40–53 for a discussion on the same. The various archaeological remains in the foothills of the eastern Himalayas belong to the various kingdoms of the Pragjyotisha-Kamrup. See L.N. Chakravarty, *Glimpses of the Early History of Arunachal*, Itanagar: Government of Arunachal Pradesh, 1995, pp. 93–103 for details on this. The British colonial accounts, however, portray a thin population in the northern banks (of the Brahmaputra) contiguous with what Arunachal today is. It is notable that the present Mishing tribe, the second-largest plain tribes of Assam after the Bodos who mostly inhabit the northern banks, are an early branch of migrants from Tibet belonging to the Abotani-tribes complex (who roughly constitute 40 per cent of the indigenous population of Arunachal today).

4. Verrier Elwin's *Democracy in NEFA*, 1965; repr., Itanagar: Government of Arunachal Pradesh, 2007, is the only work which provides an overview of the traditional polities of the frontier in one volume.
5. Verrier Elwin, *A Philosophy for NEFA*, 1957; repr., Itanagar: Government of Arunachal Pradesh, 2006, p. 8.
6. For the extent and the nature of contact through trade during the nineteenth century, see Sudatta Sikdar, 'Tribalism vs. Colonialism: British Capitalistic Intervention and Transformation of Primitive Economy of Arunachal Pradesh in the Nineteenth Century', *Social Scientist*, vol. 10, no. 12, Dec. 1982, pp. 15–31; and Sudatta Sikdar, 'Cross-Country Trade in the Making of British Policy Towards Arunachalis in the Nineteenth Century', *Proceedings of the North East India History Association* (hereafter *PNEIHA*), Second Session, Dibrugarh, 1981, pp. 210–24.
7. For details on the nature of slavery in the state see A.K. Thakur, *Slavery in Arunachal Pradesh*, New Delhi: Mittal Publications, 2003.
8. Some monographs with more intimate focus on these aspects are to be found in George Duff-Sutherland Dunbar, 'Abors and Gallongs: Notes on Certain Hill Tribes of the Indo-Tibetan Border', *Memoirs of Asiatic Society of Bengal*, vol. 5, extra no., 1915, pp. 1–91; George Duff-Sutherland Dunbar, *Other Men's Lives: A Study of Primitive Peoples*, London: Scientific Book Club, 1938; N.L. Bor, 'The Daflas and their Oaths', *Journal of the Asiatic Society of Bengal*, vol. II, no. 1, 1936, pp. 27–40; Charles R. Stonor, 'Notes on the Religion and Rituals of the Dafla Tribes of the Assam Himalayas', *Anthropos*, Bd. 52, H. 1/2. 1957, pp. 1–23; J.P. Mills, 'The Mishmis of the Lohit Valley, Assam', *The Journal of Royal Anthropological*

Institute of Great Britain and Ireland, vol. 82, no. 1, Jan.–June 1952, pp. 1–12; Christoph von Furer-Haimendorf, *Ethnographic Notes on the Tribes of the Subansiri Region*, Shillong: Assam Government Press, 1947; Idem., *Highlanders of Arunachal Pradesh*, New Delhi: Vikas Publishing House, 1982; Idem., *Himalayan Barbary*, 1955; repr. as *Himalayan Adventure*, New Delhi; Vikas Publishing House, 1983; Idem., *The Apatanis and their Neighbours: A Primitive Civilisation of the Eastern Himalayas*, London: Routledge & Kegan Paul, 1962. The authority, depth, and flair of language these monographs give to the ethnography of the Arunachali tribes are yet to be surpassed. Verrier Elwin started his 'macro-ethnography' in the 1950s and compiled a very useful volume on the nineteenth-century ethnographic writings on the tribes titled *India's North East Frontier in the Nineteenth Century*, Bombay: Oxford University Press, 1959. Among the many informative government-sponsored ethnographs on the tribes, Parul Dutta's *Aspects of Padam Minyong Culture*, 2nd edn, Itanagar: Government of Arunachal Pradesh, 1966 is held in high esteem by contemporary academics of the region.

9. Verrier Elwin, *The Art of the North-East Frontier of India*, 1959; repr., Itanagar: Government of Arunachal Pradesh, 2009, pp. 16–17.
10. K.S. Singh, ed., *People of India: Arunachal Pradesh,* vol. XIV, Calcutta: Anthropological Survey of India, 1995, pp. xiii–xiv.
11. Ibid., p. xv.
12. Retrieved from: http://www.census2011.co.in/census/state/arunachal+pradesh.html, accessed 30 March 2016.
13. Retrieved from: http://www.arunachalpradesh.gov.in/bio.htm, accessed 30 March 2016.
14. Ibid.
15. Ibid.
16. Stuart Blackburn, *Into the Hidden Valley: A Novel*, New Delhi: Speaking Tiger, 2016.
17. James Axtell, 'Ethnohistory: An Historian's Viewpoint', *Ethnohistory*, vol. 26, no. 1, Winter 1979, p. 5.
18. The terms 'pre-colonial', 'colonial', and 'post-colonial' are used for want of better terms. The use of these terms in the regional history, i.e. north-east India, has sapped the energy of the historians of the region. Examples are: David R. Syiemlieh, Presidential Address, *PNEIHA*, 31st Session, Tura, 2010, pp. 1–15; Sarah Hilaly, 'Representation of the Ethnic Communities of North-East: An Overview', *PNEIHA*, Dibrugarh, 2008, pp. 415–19; Mignonette Momin, 'Generalization in Constructing Histories

of North East India', *PNEIHA*, 24th Session, Guwahati, 2003, pp. 32–44; O.P. Kejriwal, 'The North-East in Indian Historiography: the Need for a Corrective', *PNEIHA*, 7th Session, Pasighat, 1986, pp. 17–24; Tana Showren, 'Ethnohistory in Arunachal Pradesh: Difficulties and Scope', *PNEIHA*, 27th Session, Aizawl, 2006, pp. 46–54; and Prasanta Kumar Nayak, 'History of Arunachal Pradesh: Problem of Periodization', *PNEIHA*, 28th Session, Goalpara, 2007, pp. 46–56.

19. James C. Scott, *The Art of Not Being Governed: An Anarchist History of Upland Southeast Asia*, New Haven and London: Yale University Press, 2009.
20. See Gunnel Cederlof, *Founding an Empire on India's North-Eastern Frontiers 1790–1840: Climate, Commerce, Polity*, New Delhi: Oxford University Press, 2014, pp. 235–43 for a critique of the hill–plain binary in the context of colonial expansion in north-east India.
21. Sarah Hilaly, 'Trajectory of Region Formation in the Eastern Himalayas', *Indian Historical Review*, vol. 42, no. 2, 2015, pp. 288–302.
22. Accounts of the Ahom and the British frontier policy are found in Alexander Mackenzie, *The North East Frontier of India*, 1884; repr. New Delhi: Mittal Publication, 2004; Edward Gait, *A History of Assam*, 1905, 2nd edn. 1926; repr. Delhi: Surjeet Publications, 2004, Chap. XXI, pp. 371–7; Robert Reid, *History of Frontier Areas Bordering on Assam from 1883–1941*, 1942; repr. Delhi: Eastern Publishing House, 1983; H.K. Barpujari, *Problem of the Hill Tribes: North East Frontier, 1822–42*, vol. I, Gauhati: Lawyer's Book Stall, 1970; P.N. Luthra, 'North-East Frontier Agency Tribes: Impact of Ahom and British Policy', *Economic and Political Weekly*, vol. 6, no. 23, 5 June 1971, pp. 1143–5, 1147–9; Lakshmi Devi, *Ahom-Tribal Relations: A Political Study*, Gauhati: Assam Book Depot, 1968; Bose, *History of Arunachal;* N.N. Osik, *British Relations with the Adis (1825–1947)*, New Delhi: Omsons Publications, 1992; B.N. Jha, 'British Colonial Intervention and Tribal Responses in the North East Frontier of Assam, 1825–1947', PhD diss., Arunachal University, 2002; Priyam Goswami, *The History of Assam: from Yandabo to Partition, 1826–1947*, New Delhi: Orient BlackSwan, 2012, Ch. 6. It is now common to speak of British frontier policy in Arunachal in terms of 'interventions'. A.K. Thakur's 'Processes and Agency of Precolonial States in Arunachal Pradesh', *The NEHU Journal of Social Sciences and Humanities*, vol. 1, no. 1, January 2003, pp. 1–25; and 'Socio-Economic Formations in Pre-Colonial Arunachal: Myth and Reality', *The Indian Historical Review*, vol. XXXII, no. 2, July 2005, pp. 37–63, while proposing a new and

alternate way to study pre-colonial Arunachal, do not offer views on how the 'Pre-colonial States' responded to colonial interventions.

23. Tax/blackmail/tributes levied by various, but not all, tribes on the neighbouring peasants and gold-washers of the Assam plains. The latter were subjects of the Ahom and later the colonial state. Raids were organized chiefly for extracting *posa* which was given in kind (Ahom time) and cash (British period). According to Sikdar, 'Tribalism vs Colonialism', p. 22, the reason for monetization of the posa was 'to dislodge the hill tribes from the foothills as the land was required for settlement of cultivators and for plantations'.
24. Introduced by the British in the last decades of nineteenth century, the line demarcated the operational limits of regular administration. British subjects as well as officials were not allowed to venture into or own land beyond the line without permission. It is still in force in Nagaland, Mizoram, and Arunachal Pradesh. Civil society organizations in Meghalaya and Manipur are now demanding the same to be introduced in their states.
25. John Darwin, *The Empire Project: The Rise and Fall of the British World-System, 1830–1970*, New York: Cambridge University Press, 2009, p. 1.
26. Corrupted from the title of David R. Syiemlieh, ed., *On the Edge of Empire: Four British Plans for North East India, 1941–1947*, New Delhi: Sage Publications, 2014.
27. Reid, *History of Frontier Areas*, p. 263.
28. Preamble to the Assam Frontier (Administration of Justice) Regulation, 1945, p. 1.
29. Berenice Guyot-Rechard, 'Tour Diaries and Itinerant Governance in the eastern Himalayas, 1909–1962', *The Historical Journal*, Cambridge University Press, 2017, pp. 1–24.
30. H.K. Barpujari, *American Baptist Missionaries and North East India, 1836–1900: A Documentary Study*, Gauhati: Spectrum Publications, 1986, p. lvii.
31. Andrew J. May, *Welsh Missionaries and British Imperialism: The Empire of Clouds in Northeast India*, Manchester: Manchester University Press, 2016, p. 3.
32. Rudolf Schlesinger, 'Recent Discussions on the Periodization of History', *Soviet Studies*, vol. 4, no. 2, Oct. 1952, pp. 152–69.
33. For a fuller account of tribal policy debates in India see J.N. Chaudhary, 'Post-Colonial Policy towards Ethnic Minorities of North-East India (A

Comparative Approach) with Special Reference to Arunachal Pradesh', in *Nationality, Ethnicity, and Cultural Identity in North-East India*, ed. B. Pakem, New Delhi: Omsons Publications, 1990, pp. 127–45.

34. Ramachandra Guha, *Savaging the Civilized: Verrier Elwin, His Tribals, and India*, New Delhi: Oxford University Press, 2000, p. 264.
35. Binayak Dutta, 'Constructing India's North Eastern Tribal Policy and Verrier Elwin - A Review', *PNEIHA*, 19th Session, Kohima, 1999, p. 294. A similar treatment to the subject is to be found in R.N. Prasad, 'Inner Line Regulation and its Impact on Development of North-Eastern States', in *India's North-East: The Process of Change and Development*, ed. R.K. Samanta, Delhi: B.R. Publishing Corp, 1994, pp. 89–114.
36. Betsy Taylor, 'Public Folklore, Nation-Building, and Regional Others: Comparing Apalachian USA and North-East India', *Indian Folklore Research Journal*, vol. 1, no. 2, 2002, p. 19.
37. Jawaharlal Nehru in the Foreword to Elwin, *Philosophy*.
38. Parag Chaliha, ed., *The Outlook on NEFA*, Jorhat: Asam Sahitya Sabha, 1958, p. ii.
39. S.K. Chaube, *Hill Politics in Northeast India*, 3rd edn, New Delhi: Orient Blackswan, 2012, p. 195.
40. R.K. Bhadra, and Mita Bhadra, eds., *Ethnicity, Movement and Social Structure: Contested Cultural Identity*, New Delhi: Rawat Publication, 2007, p. 2. One might debate as to how these states were 'tribal' yet the process of state formation in the North-East generally followed the ethnically tribal-rulers-getting-Hinduized pattern.
41. Tajen Dabi, 'A Nation's Begotten Child: Arunachain India's Troubled Northeast', in *Development and Ethnicity in Northeast India* eds. Komol Singha and M. Amarjeet Singh, New Delhi: Routledge, 2016, pp. 213–25.

2

Dispensaries, Doctors, and Hospitals, 1912–1950

The history of modern medicine in Arunachal goes back to the time of colonial interventions in the second decade of the twentieth century. The process gained some momentum in the mid-1940s when the ethical and institutional foundations of the health department were sought to be laid, an idea not dissimilar to the one eventually adopted and fruitfully experimented by the new government. In the wake of two important strategic considerations, the Tibetan question and World War II, the first half of the twentieth century witnessed the unprecedented use of medicine in the colonial frontier policy.

The Lost Mission: Early Christian Forays

The career of modern medicine in the hills of north-east India is generally associated with medical missions. Not surprisingly, one of the earliest references to Western medicine in Arunachal too is related to the Christian missionaries. After the Treaty of Yandaboo (1826), the American Baptist missionaries from Burma were engaged to work amongst the Singphos, Noctes, and Wanchos, the prominent eastern tribes of Arunachal. From March 1836, Nathan Brown and his team started to work first amongst the Khamptis.[1] Thereafter, the American missionaries tried to do medical work amongst the Singphos too but were not successful because of the Khampti uprising. Eventually, the objective to proselytize the Khamptis, Singphos, Noctes, and Wanchos was abandoned;[2] and the focus of the Christian mission was shifted to the Brahmaputra valley.[3]

Another phase of missionary intrusion happened in the mid-nineteenth century. In 1853, the French missionary Father Krick visited Mebo in the Siang valley and distributed medicine to the people. Krick's account reflects the missionary's belief in the superiority of Western medicine over indigenous healing and the missionary bias on the tribes' worldview. Announcing an overwhelming response to his medicine, Krick proudly reported:

> 'Yes, yes,' they all replied with one voice, 'and if you cure our sick, we shall keep you for ever, and we shall build you a house,' and in evidence of their sincerity, the chiefs put the guardhouse at my disposal. ... No sooner was I settled down in my new home than invitations poured in from all sides requesting me to go and look after the sick: being a priest, I must needs be a physician too.[4]

Like Krick, Gray was besieged by the Singphos looking for medicine.[5] These missionary explorers took interest in observing the general condition of health and disease of the people they could visit. Their medicine helped them establish friendly contact with the people who were otherwise suspicious of and often hostile to outsiders.

But for the unfavourable political circumstance (the Khampti Rebellion), the shift in focus of the mission and subsequent ban on missionary activities at the frontier, a different scenario is likely to have emerged. It is informative to remember that it was from the early twentieth century onwards that missionaries made inroads in most of today's hill states of north-east India including Nagaland and Mizoram.[6] Coincidentally, this was the period when medicine entered the lexicon of the colonial frontier policy in Arunachal.

Medicine for the Empire: Military Expeditions and Exploratory Missions

The potential threat of the Chinese in the first decades of the twentieth century led to a change in the frontier policy of the

British.[7] The murder of Noel Williamson, Assistant Political Officer, Sadiya coinciding with this changing strategic scenario, accelerated the change in British frontier policy. The Government of India executed one punitive and three political expeditions, viz., the Abor Expedition (1911–12), the Mishmi Mission (1911–12), the Miri Mission (1911–12), and the Aka Expedition (Promenade) (1913–14). The first was a punitive one while the other three were political missions.[8] Of these, the Miri Mission was the least consequential due to command and logistic flaws; the entire mission was attended by only one native hospital assistant.[9]

The origins of modern medicine in Arunachal started from this turn of events in the second decade of the twentieth century. The importance given to the health of the force as well as the medical aspect of the military expeditions is borne out by some of the reports of the above missions. Captain E.J.C. MacDonald, I.M.S., the Medical Officer of the Mishmi Mission furnished a separate medical report of the mission while Assistant Surgeon A.B. Cornelius furnished a medical report for the Nizamghat Column of the mission. Some relevant data from the same is given in Tables 2.1 (a) and 2.1 (b) below:

Table 2.1a: Disease and Casualty of the Mishmi Mission Force, 1911–12

Sl. No.	*Disease*	*Number of Cases*	*Death*
1.	Malaria	69-military; 242-Naga coolies	Nil
2.	Penumonia	2	Nil
3.	Cholera	Nil	Nil
4.	Epidemic	Nil	Nil
5.	Infectious diseases	Four isolated cases of mumps	Nil
6.	Accident	6 severe cases	1

Source: Major C. Bliss to the Inspector General of Police, Assam, Foreign Department Proceedings, Secret External, November 1912, Nos. 599–690, Appendix E, National Archives of India (NAI), New Delhi.

Table 2.1b: Diseases from which the Dacca Military Police Battalion Suffered

Sl. No.	*Disease*	*Number of Admissions*	*Percentage of Days in Hospital*
	General Diseases		
1.	Dysentery	8	.21
2.	Malaria	20	.25
3.	Rheumatic Fever	2	.02
4.	Anaemia	3	.07
	Disease of the Eye		
5.	Conjunctivitis	3	.02
6.	Corneal ulcer	2	.02
	Diseases of the Respiratory System		
7.	Bhroncitis	8	.18
	Disease of the Digestive System		
8.	Inflammation, mouth	2	.03
9.	Ditto, tonsil	3	.07
10.	Colic intestinal	2	.03
	Skin Diseases		
11.	Ringworm	1	
12.	Eczema	1	(11&12) .01
	Local Diseases		
13.	Inflammation of the Tissue	1	
14.	Abscess	2	
15.	Ulcer, leg	2	
16.	Whitlow	1	
17.	Inflammation of glands, groin	1	(local diseases) .04
	Local injuries		
18.	Abrasions, knee	1	.01
19.	Wound in hand	2	.02
20.	Wound in head	2	.01
21.	Sprain in ankle	1	.01
	Total	68	1.00

Source: Major C. Bliss to the Inspector General of Police, Assam, Foreign Department Proceedings, Secret External, November 1912, Nos. 599–690, Appendix E, NAI, New Delhi.

The detailed records of casualties and diseases of both the troops and local people underlined the importance of such military operations in generating colonial epidemiological knowledge when exploratory missions were undertaken in new frontiers. This is substantiated by the fact that Major Bliss, the Commanding Officer of the mission, made a brief note about the health status of the Mishmis and reported the prevalence of goitre, malaria, and intestinal diseases as well as opium addiction.[10] It was part of the colonial medical policy to engage doctors in acquiring knowledge about disease, places, topography, flora, and fauna during the early colonial period in India. The sense of goodwill the doctors' profession commanded was considered as the 'active agent' in the process of colonization in the newly acquired territories. The above reports show that similar measures were undertaken in Arunachal by the colonial authorities. The nature of Bliss' note reflected the same agenda. Bliss laments his inability to record the flora and fauna found in the Mishmi Hills in detail.

Bliss and Cornelius' reports served as a sort of guideline to medical challenges for subsequent military expeditions into the hills. These reports mapped the estimated risk of diseases involved in military undertakings in the hills and worked as a tentative statistical basis to counter such challenges on subsequent occasions.

Capt. G.A. Nevill's report on the Aka Promenade (1913–14) was more focused:

> The Akas and Mijis are a fairly healthy people. Goitre is very prevalent amongst them, it was noticeable that at Jamiri, where the people obtained their water from springs, there was practically no goitre. ... From enquiries it would seem that both the Akas and Mijis are gradually decreasing in numbers. This they account for as the results of epidemics of dysentery, also to the large amount of infant mortality. They apparently suffer a good deal from pneumonia during the rains.[11]

Nevill commended Captain Kennedy, the Medical Officer of the Aka mission, for the latter's 'medical work' during the mission.

Kennedy was credited as a great 'political asset in establishing good relations' with the people during the mission. It was reported that the people were willing to obtain medicine and that they made requests for dispensaries to be established in their villages. Nevill strongly recommended that such requests be acceded to since, 'it would be [by] far the easiest, cheapest, and the best way to obtain control over the country'.[12] Similar observations were made when the same mission proceeded to Tawang.

After the conclusion of operations in the Aka (Hrusso) area, Captain Nevill took an extended trip to Tawang, which was then under the effective control of the monastic Tibetan state. Captain Kennedy accompanied him taking along half a coolie load of medicine. In Tawang too, a great demand for medical relief was reported and the provisions of the visiting team proved inadequate to meet the demands of the Monpas for medicine and surgical treatment.[13] With the change in the climatic conditions, from the lower Aka (Hrusso) Hills to the great heights of Tawang, a new disease gets mentioned, viz., leprosy, which the visiting team found to be prevalent in the area. Apart from diseases, the visitors made a quick assessment of water supply, climatic conditions, and mortality.

Diseases prevalent in a particular area were not always borne in the local environment. Many were brought from outside the tribes' homesteads or from the plains. In other words, more the contact a particular group of people had with the outside world, more were the chances of getting exposed to new diseases and importing them into one's village. This was also the case with the Monpas of Tawang, who used to visit Udalguri in the Assam plains during the annual trade fair. But once in the plains, they became susceptible to diarrhoea and malaria. The promenading party came to understand this and Captain Nevill foresaw an opportunity in it: 'It would be a great boon to these folks and incidentally of considerable political value if the government were to open a dispensary at Udalguri.'[14] Aware of the importance of Udalguri trade on the Monpa livelihood, it was conceived to exploit the opportunity thrown by diarrhoea and malaria and convert it to a basis for friendly relationships with the Monpas in future.

Realizing the great potentiality of medicine, Nevill also made a more general suggestion that expeditions into hills always be accompanied by a Medical Officer along with one Sub-Assistant Surgeon (SAS) for every 30 miles of the proposed line of communication.[15] The importance urged for medical relief in frontier policy was informed by the experience in reaching out to the tribes through medicine and the positive feedback it yielded. The 'medical data' relating to the Aka Promenade as given in Table 2.2 below substantiated this view.

The below records show that medicine formed an important component of military expeditions in the hills. Diseases were a major source of suffering among the people in the hills and their reported eagerness to receive medical relief was planned to be exploited for diplomatic and political ends. In the Arunachal hills, medicine did not merely serve the military but it was carefully envisaged to be an important and integral part of the policy of extending political influence in the un-administered hills. For this to become successful, it was important to have some sort of medical infrastructure set up in the hills.

The military outposts left behind by the expeditionary forces in the hills became the first emblem of this policy. It was from one such outpost that on 29 April 1912, Captain E.C.J. McDonald, who had earlier served the Mishmi Mission as the medical officer, was appointed the first medical officer for the Balek outpost in Pasighat.[16] Before this, the military surgeon at Sadiya took up cases of fracture of limbs, eye diseases, and the like brought into the station by the neighbouring hill tribes.[17]

Meanwhile, the government introduced some administrative changes as part of administrative re-organization to have more

Table 2.2: Patients Treated during the Aka Promenade, 1913–14

Diseases	*No. of Monpa Patients*	*No. of Aka Patients*	*No. of Nyishi Patients*	*Remarks*
Abscess	4	1	–	
Asthma	2	–	–	
Bronchitis	4	11	4	
Colic (intestinal)	3	–	–	
Carious tooth	2	–	–	Extracted
Debility	6	4	–	
Diarrhoea	3	–	–	
Diseases of the digestive system	5	12	–	
Diseases of the heart	1	–	–	
Diseases of the ear	–	1	–	
Diseases of the eye	5	5	2	
Diseases of the nerve	3	–	–	
Diseases of the skin	1	–	1	
Dislocation	–	–	1	Hip
Dyspepsia	2	4	1	
Fevers	5	6	–	
Fly-bite ulcer	–	1	–	
Fracture	1	–	1	
Goitre	1	44	34	
Gonorrhoea	1	–	–	
Malaria	15	–	–	
Myalgia	–	–	1	
Pneumonia	2	–	–	
Rheumatism	3	8	6	
Syphilis	1	–	–	
Sprain	–	3	–	
Ulcer	1	15	5	
Wound	6	6	6	
Worms	3	–	–	
Total	80	123	63	265

Source: 'Report by Capt. G.A. Nevill on the Aka Promenade, 1913–14', Foreign and Political Department Proceedings, Secret E, April 1915, Nos. 64–6, Part I, pp. 8, 10, NAI, New Delhi.

effective control of the North-East Frontier (NEF). In October 1912, the tract to the east of Subansiri was placed under the charge of Dundas with headquarters at Sadiya, and the tract west of Subansiri was placed under Nevill who was to be under the direct supervision of the Chief Commissioner (of Assam).[18] It was at this stage that the appointment of McDonald at Balek outpost was done as part of what was termed in official parlance as the 'control of the North-East Frontier'.[19] The appointment of McDonald was made against the creation of a temporary post of second-class Civil Surgeon (CS) for six months on 1 August 1912.[20] The pay of the CS was borne from the imperial government exchequer and not from provincial revenue.[21]

On 16 October 1912, the Government of India, Foreign Department sanctioned a permanent Indian Medical Service (IMS) post for the Dibrugarh Frontier through which the service of McDonald was extended.[22] One post of Military Assistant Surgeon (MAS) and three Sub-Assistant Surgeons (SASs) were also sanctioned for the NEF, the actual appointments and posting being subject to specific requirements at subsequent stages.[23] E.G. Crunden (MAS Class III) was appointed as the medical officer at Sadiya on 7 July 1913.[24] He was originally supposed to be posted at the outposts in Lohit valley once the construction of roads and occupation of the outpost were completed.[25] It is to be noted that the above posts were military and, under the rules prevalent at the time, only Europeans were eligible for appointment to these posts.

The creation of medical posts and appointments of doctors was part of a plan for a type of medical administration meant for all the outposts in NEFT. A correspondence made on 7 July 1912 between the Commissioner of Assam and the Foreign Department, Government of India clearly stated about establishing 'gradual control over the North-East Frontier'.[26] The medical budget of the plan is shown in Table 2.3 below.

Table 2.3: Estimate of the Cost of Control of the North-East Frontier, 1912

Particulars	*Monthly Cost in Rupees*	*Annual Cost in Rupees*
Medical Officer	550	6,600
Local allowance for Medical Officers	200	2,400
Military Assistant Surgeon	250	3,000
Local allowance for Military Assistant Surgeon	100	1,200
Three Sub-Assistant Surgeons at Rs.40	120	1,440
Local allowances for three Sub-Assistant Surgeons at Rs.20	60	720

Source: Kennedy to the Secretary, the Secretary to the Govt. of India, File No. M.O./12 (M) of 1914, Assam Secretariat, Municipal Department, Medical-A, March 1914, Nos. 3–11, SAGAP, State Archives, Government of Arunachal Pradesh, Itanagar.

The bright prospect of medical as a discreet arm of colonial intervention soon attracted attention at the right corners; Archdale Earle, the Chief Commissioner of Assam, outlined the policy thus: 'It is extremely important that we should press on medical and educational schemes, but particularly medical schemes, in the newly acquired areas. Medical relief is most urgently required, and it will be the most important way in which we shall get into touch with the wild tribes.'[27]

Towards this end, expansion of medical establishments was planned and some sanitary measures were also initiated. In 1915, the outpost hospital at Balek (Pasighat) was enlarged with provisions for indoor patients.[28] One of the earliest challenges of the hospital was the menace of malaria. In 1918, anti-malarial measures were carried out under the direction of the Sanitary Commissioner and a sum of Rs.300 was incurred in connection with the anti-malarial measures.[29] Birendra Nath Sen Gupta (AS) and Ghute Gurung, the peon were commended for their work with a reward of Rs.20 each.

The 'medical thrust' on the NEFT was so important that even when fiscal austerity was advocated for regular provinces of the empire, the same was not applied at the frontier. In 1923, the Bengal Retrenchment Committee Report suggested a reduction of medical expenditure in the Brahmaputra valley.[30] But the recommendations were not applied in the case of medical expenditure for the frontier areas. The sanctioned cadre of the Indian Medical Service (IMS) in Assam comprised twelve officers plus two officers as leave reserve; of these fourteen officers, one served as the Civil Surgeon (CS) of the Sadiya Frontier Tract. Out of the seven MAS employed in Assam in 1923, one was Mr Gloria, posted as Assistant Surgeon at Pasighat and the other was Lieutenant Mullins, a Civil Surgeon at Sadiya headquarters.[31]

The four exploratory missions had established the actual extent of the alleged Chinese/Tibetan influence in the frontier. The Abor Expedition and the Miri Mission did not find any trace of the Tibetan or Chinese influence except some contacts in the extreme north of the Adi areas.[32] But since the Mishmi Mission confirmed the prevailing strategic anxiety, the situation in the Mishmi area was deemed urgent: road construction leading to the proposed border military outpost at Walong and other places considered important in the Lohit Valley was thus started.[33] Called the Lohit Valley Road Project, this was the first major infrastructure project undertaken in the entire NEFT before World War II. It is not a mere coincidence that the country's largest river bridge has come up in the same region recently. The British might have left the Brahmaputra valley; strategic worries have not.

The Sadiya Civil Hospital

Sadiya was the easternmost strategically important military-administrative outpost of the East India Company (EIC) since the end of the first Burmese war (1826). Located at the crossroads of

Burma, Tibet, and India, and in the confluence of the Siang (Tsangpo), Dibang, and Lohit rivers, it was the outpost from where the affairs of the Khamptis and the Singphos (in the nineteenth century), and later on the Mishmis and the Adis (in the nineteenth and the twentieth centuries), were managed—first through military expeditions, and from the last decade of the nineteenth century, through an assistant political officer. The outpost emerged to be an important administrative and thriving trade centre where the tribesmen regularly flocked to receive, and spend, their monetized *posa*, as well as sell their goods and make purchases. Given the stated policy of the use of medicine in frontier diplomacy since the early twentieth century, it was obvious that healthcare acquired an important component in the teeming town's infrastructure plan.

Originally built in 1914, the hospital at Sadiya had two small wards made of wood and bamboo capable of hosting twelve male patients and four female patients at a time.[34] A separate dispensary made of bamboo near the river dealt largely with the coolie corps. Because of encroachment in 1922, the hospital was moved to a site nearer the town. The basic provisions of the hospital and the working conditions of the staff were reported to be worse. The Civil Surgeon appraised the government:

> To the staff, work under such conditions fails to convey the impression that it is a seriously meant effort to cope with the medical requirements of a large virgin district. If medicine is to acquire the importance which is desirable in a political district, in the first instance let us raise our standard of work and housing at headquarters, where treatment is more thorough and cures proportionately more lasting.[35]

And the coveted service the hospital was supposed to render to the empire's interest can be seen from the comments of Lt. Colonel H. Innes, the Officiating Inspector-General of Civil Hospitals, (IGCH) Assam:

Medical relief is a great asset from a political point of view and [a] large number of hill people come in to Sadiya for treatment, many from great distances. To-day a Lama from Thibet hearing of the fame of the hospital has come for treatment and there is no doubt the present buildings are an eye sore and in no way worthy of the British Raj not only are they unsuitable but they are costly to maintain and the time has come to do something better ... what is wanted here is a young active officer prepared to devote himself to medical and surgical work, to learn to speak the language and to realise his responsibilities as a civilizing influence.[36]

To improve and expand the hospital, a proposal amounting to Rs.71,130 for the cost of renovation was sent to the Government of India with the following justification: 'The civilizing influence of a well-administered hospital on the various tribes who visit Sadiya is remarkable, but at present, the condition of the buildings is such as to discourage attendance.'[37] The visual impact the hospital building could have on the perception of the visiting tribes was one of the concerns of the ICGH; the conviction that the grandeur of the Raj, to be reflected in the imposing architectural marvel of the Sadiya hospital, was not entirely misplaced in a region where the local architecture was primarily based on bamboo huts and thatched roofs, and where the hospitals and dispensaries were the first civic institutions of the empire to be frequented by the tribes. Table 2.4 shows the work of the hospital for a three-year period while Table 2.5 shows its budget for the year 1925.

Besides the refurbishment of the Sadiya hospital, the dilapidated dispensary at Denning in the Lohit valley, originally a Public Work Department (PWD) dispensary meant for the coolies working in the Lohit Valley Road Project, was considered for revival as a part of the 'forward policy' in the valley in the wake of the confirmed Tibetan influence. Accordingly, an amount of Rs.27,241 was sanctioned for its restoration and renovation.[38] Unlike the Sadiya hospital, the service put in by the Denning dispensary pleased the Governor of Assam: 'The Sub-Assistant

Table 2.4: Patients Treated in the Sadiya Civil Hospital during 1924, 1925, and 1927

Year	*Outpatient (daily average)*	*In-Patient/ Indoor*	*Operations Performed*	*Remarks*
1924	18.75	13.48	19 major including 4 cataracts	Figures for 1927 reflect a total of the year. Average NA
1925	15.24	15.22	15 with 5 cataracts	
1927	3,271	261	NA	

Source: The figures for the years 1924 and 1925 are derived from the inspection remarks by Lt. Col. Innes, IGCH dated 19 Jan. 1926, and that of 1927 from the inspection remarks by the Governor of Assam on the hospital dated 31 Jan. 1928, Assam Secretariat, Medical-A, March 1928, No. 70, pp. 3–5, SAGAP, Itanagar.

Table 2.5: Budget of the Sadiya Civil Hospital for the Year 1925

Total Receipt (in Rupees)	*Expense Sub-Head (in Rupees)*		
	Staff Salaries and Pay of Assistant Surgeon	*Establishment*	*Medicines*
Total= 11,089-13-3 including Subscriptions: Europeans = 60 Indians = 240	5,017	1,523	4,218

Source: Inspection remarks of IGCH dated 19 Jan. 1926, Assam Secretariat, Medical-A, March 1928, No. 70, p. 3, SAGAP, Itanagar.

Surgeon appears to be doing good work. He should do all he can to win the confidence of the hill tribes.'[39]

How strategic necessity shaped the colonial medical policy can be gauged from the fact that the outpost dispensary in the Siang valley started in 1912 was not extended beyond the foothill station of Pasighat because the suspected Tibetan influence in the area was found to be a false alarm. Instead, the focus shifted to the Lohit valley where the influence was perceived to be inimical to imperial strategic considerations. Thus, the dispensary at Pasighat, unlike that of Sadiya hospital and the Denning dispensary, was strengthened only for the needs of the Assam Rifles (AR): the jungle was cleared in 1919 to check the spread of malaria for which a special grant of Rs.5,000 was spent;[40] and, there was a new water supply scheme amounting to a sum of Rs.8,000.[41]

On the whole, the decades before World War II witnessed the strategic employment of medicine, doctor, and dispensary in the Siang and Lohit valleys of the Sadiya Frontier Tract.

Plans for the Balipara Frontier Tract

The developments in the Kameng and Subansiri valleys of the Balipara Frontier Tract convey the same strategic considerations in the question of opening dispensaries. The Miri Mission did not find any instance of Tibetan intrusion in the area. As a result, the same level of urgency to introduce and improvise dispensaries and hospitals to attract people, as witnessed in Lohit and Sadiya, did not happen. However, as a general index to frontier policy, medicine continued to be written in bold letters.

In the year 1921, the administrative headquarters of the Balipara Frontier Tract was transferred to Charduar after the 5th Battalion of the AR was formed in 1920 with its headquarters at Lokra.[42] In the same year, a post of Civil Assistant Surgeon (CAS) was established and attached to the AR Battalion and its cost was debited to the Provincial Revenue.[43] In 1930, the CAS was placed under the general supervision of the CS, Darrang, and the pay and allowances of the officer were debited to the Central Revenue.[44] Subsequently, owing to administrative inconvenience, the CAS was placed in subordinate medical charge of the Tract under the general supervision of the CS, Darrang, who also doubled as the acting CS of the Tract.

In 1932, after the 5th Battalion of the AR at Lokra was amalgamated with the 2nd Battalion of the AR at Sadiya, the post of the CAS was done away with and the medical work of the area was placed under the direct charge of the CS, Darrang. The latter was expected to tour the administered territories twelve times a year and a fixed contribution of Rs.1,200 per annum from the Central to the Provincial Revenue towards the pay and travelling allowance related to this was made.[45]

It is notable that the amalgamated battalion of the AR was shifted from Lokra to Sadiya (along with the withdrawal of the post of CAS). This sits perfectly with the increased strategic concerns in the eastern sector (Lohit valley) vis-à-vis the Tibetan influence. At the same time, the special allowance made to the CS, Darrang, shows that a sort of 'medical administration' was kept in reserve for the western sector (Balipara Frontier Tract) to woo the Monpas just in case the Tibetans showed up unexpectedly.

The financial component too was meagre as compared to the eastern sector. The total estimate of expenditure on health for the year 1926 was Rs.9,900 (non-recurring) and Rs.1,675 (recurring) of which the latter mostly comprised the payments of one SAS, one vaccinator, medicine, etc.[46] These staff belonged to the hospital at Charduar and Lokra, the headquarters of the Political Officer and the battalion of the AR (till 1932) respectively. These medical establishments in the administrative and military centres in the foothills became the base for sporadic yet politically fruitful medical work in the interior villages of the hills of the extensive Balipara frontier.

The interest shown by the Nyishi, Aka (Hrussa), and the Monpas in medical relief was one of the major highlights of the Aka Promenade and the Tawang Expedition (1913–14). Captain G.A. Nevill, who eventually served as the Political Officer of the Balipara frontier from 1919 to 1928, in his administrative report for the year 1924–5 mentioned that when an exploratory team visited the Aka (Hrusso) area in February 1925, a petition was made by the people for the establishment of a dispensary in their country, a request first made to the same officer during the Aka Promenade ten years ago. Captain Nevill made a strong recommendation for a dispensary led by a good and competent SAS to be established in the Aka (Hrusso) area.[47]

It is evident that people were attracted to the palliative effects of medicine and the frontier officials were too happy to cash in on this positive impression. For instance, Captain Nevill in his administrative report for the year 1927–8 states that 'the Akas and the Nyishis had gradually gained confidence and were becoming appreciative of the benefits of the new order'.[48] Nevill suggested a small garrison with a British officer, a dispensary and a Sub-Assistant Surgeon to be attached to every post in the frontier, 'as' he pejoratively justifies, 'a hospital for treatment of sickness is appreciated by the savage more than anything else'.[49] It is important to note that the above suggestions were made after the Ranganadi (Panyor) Expedition on the eastern Nyishis in 1926–7 after which four places in the Balipara frontier were identified for the establishment of military outposts with dispensaries attached to each of them. Table 2.6 illustrates this emerging strategy.

On 21 May 1928, R.C.R. Cumming succeeded Captain Nevill as the Political Officer who, in turn, followed up some of Nevill's proposals. It was planned to construct a road in the Aka area with a cold-weather outpost and a dispensary at Jamiri.[50] The total amount of the project, consisting of one SAS, one compounder, one sweeper, and medicine, was estimated at Rs.2,190 and a separate sum of Rs.750 for the purchase of medicine to be distributed amongst the tribes. Another proposal for a sum of Rs.3,916 was also submitted to the Imperial Government for improving the Charduar Dispensary to cater to the increasing demands for medicine.[51] Records on the actual implementation of the above proposals are sketchy but the proposals by themselves underline the importance of medicine attached to the frontier policy.

The overall amount spent on medical and healthcare facilities

Table 2.6: Nevill's Proposal for Dispensaries in Balipara Frontier Tract, 1928

Place (arranged in order of importance Nevill placed to each) and its Strategic importance		*Remarks*
Jamiri (in the Aka area)	Located strategically between the Akas, the Mijis, the Nyishis, and the Mompas of Rupa-Shergaon. The latter was located en route Bhutan and the trade route to Udalguri fair.	The Jamiri dispensary was opened in 1928–9, abandoned in 1930–1
The Apatani country	As a base for controlling the 'turbulent' Ranganadi valley	
Miripathar	As a base to control the Nyishi area east of Bhorelli and west of Poma	
Dikrang valley	As a base to control the Nyishi area east of Miripathar; sparsely populated 'owing to the state of anarchy that has existed' here for many years past.	

Source: The data appearing in the table has been derived from Reid, *History of the Frontier Areas*, pp. 292–3. Words in quotation marks are those of Reid.

in the Sadiya and the Balipara frontier tracts from 1921–2 to 1925–6 is shown in Table 2.7 below.

Table 2.7: Expenditure on Medical and Public Health during the Year 1921–6

Head of Scheme	*1921–2*	*1922–3*	*1923–4*	*1924–5*	*1925–6*	*Total*
	Rs.	*Rs.*	*Rs.*	*Rs.*	*Rs.*	*Rs.*
Medical	52,462	46,719	50,418	51,616	52,288	2,53,503
Public Health	1,024	1,090	1,289	1,536	1,870	6,809
Total	53,486	47,089	51,707	53,152	54,158	2,59,592

Source: Abridged from Soames to Foreign Secretary to the Government of India dated 19 January 1927, Assam Secretariat, Medical-B, June 1928, Nos. 109–115, File No. PH/706, Statement II, SAGAP, Itanagar.

The total expenditure in Manipur for the same period was about Rs.38,333.[52] On the whole, in the first twenty-five years since the 'opening' of the North-East Frontier (1911–12) medical relief became the chief instrument of the public seduction of the tribes whose relationship with the colonial state in the nineteenth century was marked by recurrent hostility and fragile truce.

Wartime Dispensaries: The First Anthropologist at the Frontier

The next phase of the frontier officials' engagement with the NEFT tribes and express use of medicine to back it up happened in the wake of World War II. The intervening period, roughly from 1915 to 1938, was described by G.E.D. Walker, Political Officer, Sadiya Frontier Tract as a period of 'complete blackout', a time when there was 'limited intercourse' between the administration and the hills tribes of the NEFT.[53] The threat of Japan in the North-East had compelled the government to pursue a policy of 'gradual penetration', that is to speed up direct administrative control of the NEFT. Under this scheme, in 1943, Mr J.P. Mills, the veteran administrator of the Naga Hills, was appointed as the Adviser to the Governor of Assam for Tribal Areas.[54] In the same year, the Tirap Frontier Tract was created under a separate Political Officer for administrative convenience in the war efforts. For the same reasons, in 1946, the Balipara Frontier Tract was divided into two administrative units, viz., the Sela Sub-Agency (Kameng region) and the Subansiri Area.

Expansion of dispensaries was initiated during this phase and medical relief reached further in some of the strategically located interior villages: at Karko (1940), Riga (1940), and Pangin (1945) in the Siang valley and Rupa (1943) and Dirangdzong (1944) in the Monpa region. In the Lohit valley, a small medical team was already attached to the Lohit Valley Road Project.[55] In January

1945, the Government of India sanctioned two posts of SAS, two compounders, two peons, and two medicine carriers for the Lohit Valley Road Project being executed by the Central Public Work Department (CPWD).[56] It has already been noted that this road project was part of the policy to check Tibetan influence in the Lohit valley. In the Tirap Frontier Tract, many ad hoc dispensaries were set up along the Stilwell Road during World War II. These were located at various places: Tipangpani, north Tirap, Namchik, Kumlao, and Hell Gate; all of these were closed as soon as the war was over.[57] As on October 1945, the sanctioned strength of doctors in Tirap was two SAS, who were posted at Lonke and Khonsa.[58]

In February 1944, Christoph von Furer-Haimendorf was appointed as the Special Officer of the newly designated Subansiri Area making him by default the first individual colonial officer to have been formally sent far inside the Subansiri hills beyond the Inner Line. As if a lesson was derived from this fact, the Nehru government later also appointed an anthropologist (Verrier Elwin) to steer the newly created NEFA administration. The Austrian anthropologist shared Walker's view that no effective steps or exploratory operations were carried out in the (Subansiri) region after the Miri Mission.[59] Furer-Haimendorf 's assigned job was exploratory, not of establishing political control but a reconnoitring one. During his three trips to the area ably assisted by his wife Betsy, he was accompanied by Assistant Surgeon Dr Bhattacharjee and a compounder.[60] It requires no depth of poetic imagination that the Rockefeller scholar[61] and Adviser to the Governor of Assam J.P. Mill's friend, who is still the foremost authority on the Subansiri tribes, and brought one of it, the Apatanis, to the coffee table of anthropologists worldwide, must have made good use of medical relief just as he did with his fieldwork methods and tools.

Mr J.P. Mills, the Adviser to the Governor of Assam on Tribal

Affairs visited Ziro, the Apatani valley in 1945. While lamenting over the condition of the dispensary and the doctors' quarters at Duta, he said that medical relief was eagerly sought by the tribesmen and that a good 'field' exists for medical work in the area.[62] As fate would have had it that way, Mills lost his daughter Phillipa, who had accompanied her father, to a fever contracted during the tour before she could be evacuated to a hospital in the plains.[63] Mill's concern for medical amenities in Subansiri turned out to be ominous; the lack of it cost him his own daughter. If a local fellow's opinion was sought on this, the personal misfortune of the able officer would have been identified to be the Yapoms' (sylvan deities) handiwork. The gods having taken a prized *yudum* (sacrificial offerings, usually animals, made to the gods), it was time for the government to appropriately tame the mountains.

In October 1946, Major F.N. Betts was appointed the first Political Officer of the Subansiri Area with the task of establishing a headquarters.[64] Young and fresh from the World War II campaign in the Burma theatre, Major Betts was accompanied by an anthropologically bent wife Ursula whose memoir rivals that of Furer-Haimendorf and Elwin.[65] Atop the new headquarters established at Kore, the Union Jack proudly oversaw the neighbouring Nyishi villages.[66] Around the same time, W.J.L. Neal, the CS, visited the area and reported about the health situation and proposed expansion of administrative and medical measures. The existing facilities and Neal's plan are given in Table 2.8 below.

There was no hospital building at Kore, the headquarters of the Political Officer, and neither was there any dispensary in Ziro plateau. It was reported that diseases like malaria, which were contracted during visits to the plains in Assam, were prevalent in the area. Diseases of the respiratory tract, skin, and goitre were also reported.

Table 2.8: Medical Situation in Subansiri, 1946

KORE-HQ of the P.O.	*Neal's Medical Plan*	*Existing Sanctioned Medical Staff*
Political Officers' Bungalow	A hospital at Base (Dejoo?)	One Assistant Surgeon at Kore
5th Assam Rifles' detachment Accommodation for 25	Hospital for 5th Assam Rifles & PLCs at Yatchouli	One Sub-Assistant Surgeon at Yatchouli (on leave)
Interpreter's quarters	A Hospital at KORE (Headquarters of P.O.)	One Sub-Assistant Surgeon, itinerating (not filled)
Some staff quarters		
Political Godown		
Assistant Surgeon's quarter	A Dispensary in the Apa Tani Country	Two compounders

Source: Derived from the Inspection remarks by the Political Officer, Balipara Frontier Tract, Medical Department, Medical Branch, File No. 24/20 of 1945, SAGAP, Itanagar.

Medical Tours and Treating a Bhutanese Official

With the expansion of dispensaries, another fixture was added in the relationship between the people and the colonial authorities—the annual tours of the medical officers in the interior villages.

On 28 February 1945, the Dirangdzong Dispensary was inspected by I. Ali, Political Officer of the Balipara Frontier Tract, a year after it was opened.[67] Ali's inspection report is a valuable account of the functioning of dispensaries and the efficacy of medical diplomacy in tribal areas in general. One Lt. Thantluanga was in charge of the dispensary assisted by Azizur Rahman, the compounder; both of whom were found to be doing 'excellent work'. The total number of patients treated within a year was about 7,108 and those administered with vaccination 8,023. Goitre and malaria were common ailments. Villages settled nearby the outpost were visited frequently and distant ones were visited once a month. The doctor was generally accompanied by the AR personnel during the tours. This practice of taking military escort during health tours in villages was criticized by Ali who considered that the service of an interpreter in place of the military escort would be more rewarding.

Medical tours with military escort in an unadministered, internally restive hills, ever suspicious of outsiders, is understood but the idea of engaging interpreters in place of military escorts speaks two important things—that people were receptive to medical relief and that the policy of using medicine in frontier policy was bearing fruit. The initial investment made in winning the confidence of the people now generated the confidence to tread the interior villages in the hills with medicine alone, without arms.

At around the same time, the Dirang Dzong outpost dispensary medical officer, Lt. Thantluanga, was confronted by a messenger from the syphilis-stricken Tashigong Dzongpen of Bhutan requesting immediate treatment.[68] Being a case from an 'international' patient, the matter was referred to the Political Officer at Charduar who promptly authorized treatment. The justification given by the Political Officer was that it was important to help the friendly Dzongpen to maintain the post at Dirang Dzong.[69] The Dzongpen had earlier supplied the outpost at Dirang Dzong with 150 mounds of rice at a low price and, in the estimation of the Political Officer, the Dzongpen's goodwill was crucial to long term imperial interest in the Monpa area where Tibetan officials continued to collect taxes at the time.

Epidemics, Blockades, and Medical Relief

In 1935, an outbreak of the smallpox epidemic was reported from the hills beyond Denning in Lohit valley in March at Chowkham in the Khampti area in April, and at Mime-Sipo in Siang in May. By July, about 100 deaths were reported from Chongkham, Munglang, Latao, and Mumong in the Khampti areas.[70] The epidemic spread to the unadministered Mishmi area in the north wherefrom people regularly came down to Sadiya for trade. This posed a threat to the health of the strategically important administrative outpost.

A vaccinator and a guard were placed at the Deopani crossing to ensure that people coming from infected Mishmi areas were vaccinated and no infected cases entered Sadiya. Orders were issued by which Adis and Mishmis were prevented from entering Sadiya unless they were vaccinated. In response to this order, a deputation of Adis from Dambuk and Bomjur villages requested for a vaccinator to be sent to their areas. W.H. Calvert, the Political Officer, who received the petition, commented that the perception of the people was different a few years back when it was not uncommon for government vaccinators to be chased out from their village.[71] The above order, which required compulsory vaccination before entering Sadiya, was like steps taken in the nineteenth century when infected coolies from Bengal embarked at Assam ports. Epidemics, along with raids, had become a legitimate excuse for raising blockades on the tribes.

Some emergency medical reliefs during epidemics were also undertaken during the period. The urgency and dedication with which the relief measures were carried out bear testimony to the frontier administrations' object to find a warm spot in the hearts of the people through aid and relief. In July 1945, the dysentery epidemic affected the Adi villages of Koni-Yogeng, Simong, Riga, Pareng, Yeksing, Pangin, and Rotung on the right bank of Siang.[72] Relief was immediately provided and, as a result, no casualty was reported. A similar epidemic gripped Lohit valley in September 1946. The data on the epidemic is given in Table 2.9.

It can be seen from the table that medical relief was provided in a reasonably quick manner, as a result of which about two-thirds of the patients were saved.

Malaria was one of the graveyards of the early colonial explorers in the tropics. The foothills of Arunachal were no different in

Table 2.9: Dysentery Epidemic in Lohit, 1946

Affected Villages	*Disease*	*Date of Outbreak*	*Date of Reporting*	*Date of Medical Relief Provided*	*Total no. of Cases*	*Total no. of Deaths*	*Total no. of cured*	*Remarks*
Neyanglat Sangunlat Walenglat Walaglat, Kamdiglat Blonglat Slonglat Kamlalglat	Bacillary Dysentery Dysentery	First week of July 1946	28-06-48	11-09-46	95	33	62	Medical Officer I/C Walong outpost visited the affected areas and distributed medicines

Source: Abridged from File No. 129/29 of 1946, Medical Department, NEFA Branch, SAGAP, Itanagar.

this regard. Anti-malarial measures, earlier undertaken in the AR outpost at Pasighat, were renewed there and at Charduar during the years 1945–7. Standard manuals on the control of malaria like that of Brigadier G. Covell's *Anti-Mosquito Measures: With Special Reference to India* were consulted and all necessary steps were adopted.[73] In Charduar and Lokra, an anti-malaria expert Major Kar, Assistant Director of Public Health (Malariology) in the Provincial Government of Assam was entrusted to make an investigation and submit a comprehensive report on the matter, a part of which is given in Table 2.10.

The AR men regularly fell sick soon after coming back from tours in the hills. Sadiya, as noted earlier, already had a relatively better hospital to look after the eastern sector. Pasighat was emerging as an important administrative outpost after the Abor Expedition (1911–12); this arrangement took care of affairs between the Lohit-Dibang valleys in the east and Subansiri in the west, at least near the foothills. Charduar remained the base for

Table 2.10: Malaria cases in Charduar dispensary and the 5th Assam Rifles Hospital, Lokra

Year	*Charduar Dispensary*	*Assam Rifles Hospitals, Lokra*
1944	160	NA
1945	245	277
1946	192	81
1947	166	236
1948	202	520

Source: Abridged from Office of the Adviser to the Governor of Assam on Tribal Areas, File No. Med- 45/48 of 1948, SAGAP, Itanagar.

Subansiri and Kameng (Sela) region; the health of the AR posted in the tract was too important a matter to be left to alleviative medical interventions. Thus, more serious measures were resorted to when required in the military stations, unlike those in the hills where the arrangement was minimal, expedient, and transitory.

Reforms in Medical Administration

By July 1946, the total sanctioned medical staff for the tribal areas of NEFA (as separate from those meant for the AR) was one CS, four AS, fourteen SAS, and seventeen compounders.[74] But the actual strength was five AS and seven SAS.[75] Of these, four Assistant Surgeons were from the Indian Army Medical Corps (IAMC) and the remaining one from the Assam Provincial Cadre while five SAS were from the AR and two were exclusively sanctioned for the Agency.[76]

The prevalent system of fixed dispensaries limited the scope of using medicine to influence people in the interior areas despite occasional tours that were undertaken. Also, medical tours were reported to be unsuitable for the medical staff serving in the interior outposts, most of whom were recruited from the plains and were unable to cope with prolonged residence in the hills.[77] Away from family and civilization, they suffered from psychological problems.[78] One Dr Dutta, in charge of Lonke Dispensary in Tirap, died in an apparent case of suicide resulting from loneliness.[79] Numerous complaints of inconveniences, loneliness, and requests for transfer were regularly reported after more dispensaries were opened in the interior villages. Lack of communication, proper accommodation, and rationing along with the absence of a transfer policy added to their woes. This was a new challenge in the medical administration before the government.

The medical administration of NEFA was under the general supervision of the IGCH, Assam, with the Civil Surgeon at Sadiya assumed to be in the field. As discussed earlier, the Civil Surgeon, Darrang, was in nominal charge of the medical affairs of the Balipara frontier. The justification for this arrangement was the vast geographical expanse of the frontier.

The existing system of medical administration suffered from two defects, viz., lack of proper supervision of medical works in the hills because of the vast geographical expanse of the frontier and the anomalous position of medical staff. Two classes of doctors were posted in the hills—one for the Assam Rifles and another for the tribes—with different scales of pay and service conditions.[80] It was proposed to bring about a uniform system of medical administration in place of the existing one which was confusing and anomalous. Standardization of medical administration became imminent and a separate cadre of medical service for the frontier was sought to be created.

Reforms of varying degrees were advocated. The following measures adopted in the Tirap Frontier Tract are indicative of the broader medical reforms on the anvil:

1. Strengthening of the Base Hospital (Margherita) in a fairly well-equipped condition with about thirty beds.
2. Itinerating doctors, two or three in number, to tour around the

villages with suitable drugs, viz., Mepacrine sulph drugs, laxative tablets, A.P.C. tablets, vitamin tablets, ointments, eye drops, etc.).

3. Their duties will be:
   (a) to distribute medicines to the sick;
   (b) to select cases that need hospitalization;
   (c) to arrange to send them to Base Hospital;
   (d) propaganda work;
   (e) preaching sanitation; and,
   (f) other health measures.
4. The doctors should be supplied with camp comforts and arrangements, and stay in each village for two, three, or four days as they think necessary and return to the headquarters after a month or two for rest, refilling the spent stock, and submission of reports with comments.
5. Each one of them may be in charge of the Base Hospital for some time in turn.
6. Dispensaries and hospitals can be established by gradually watching the response and result of this system in suitable places.
7. If doctors to do such work are not available, a start can be made even with compounders and trained Rural Health Inspectors.[81]

These proposals were accepted and the construction of a Base Hospital at Margherita, the headquarters of the Political Officer, began.

Among the broader steps proposed were: construction of family quarters for the medical staff; to take over the Civil Hospitals at Charduar and Pasighat by the Agency (NEFA) administration from the provincial government of Assam; to pay the doctors from the 'Agency Budget'; to grant two months' leave in a year to the staff; and, to make ration provisions. These reform proposals made by the CS, Sadiya, were recommended by Lt. Col. E.T.N. Taylor, the IGCH, Assam, to the Government of India with these solemn words: 'I know of no better way of "showing the flag" than that of providing good modern medical treatment in hills areas.'[82]

The proposed reforms were planned to cover all possible locations in the frontier considered important from military and strategic points of view (see Appendix I). The farthest outposts like Dirangzong, Kirum, Walong, and Punging were meant to be base outposts from where itinerating doctors were supposed to accompany the Political Officer during tours to the interior villages. It was reflected in the proposal that the hospitals were meant to be set up in places alongside the military outposts. The underlying rationale behind this step must have been to present the military outposts as a symbol of medical relief rather than a military bastion ready to infringe upon the tribes' independence. The hospitals so established were supposed to look after the health of both the Assam Rifles personnel and the native population. In remote places where the posting of a doctor was not possible, it was planned to post a compounder. The work of these hospitals was to be controlled and coordinated by larger hospitals designated as 'Base Hospitals' located at the four foothill stations, namely Charduar and Joyhing for the western section, and Pasighat and Sadiya for the eastern, under a separate Civil Surgeon in each.

The fund for materializing the proposed expansion and reform was one of the concerns of the Government of India. To save cost, it was suggested to amalgamate the Agency and the Assam Rifles doctors into one cadre with an outpost allowance for the doctors instead of looking after the Assam Rifles. The Ministry of External Affairs, Government of India, while discussing the proposal, agreed that good medical attention was the key to secure the goodwill of the tribesmen and establishment of government influence.[83] On 8 April 1946, the Governor-General-in-Council temporarily sanctioned the constitution of a combined medical cadre for the Agency as shown in Table 2.11.

Further, four posts of medicine carriers at Rs. 35 and five peons at Rs.35 each per month with special pay were subsequently sanctioned to the amalgamated cadre.

Table 2.11: Medical Cadre for NEFA, 1946

Category of Post	*No. of Posts*	*Pay*
Assistant Surgeons	4	Rs.150–160–20/2–300–25/2–400 P.M. each for Provincial Medical Service Officer or rank pay for an Indian Army Medical Corps Officer
Sub-Assistant Surgeons	14	Rs.75–5–175 P.M. each
Compounders	17	Rs.30–1–40 P.M. each

Source: Under Secretary to the Government of India to the Secretary to the Governor of Assam, Memo No. F. 14 (9)-E/45, Assam Governor's Secretariat, Military Secretary's Office, 1945, File No. A 1045/56, SAGAP, Itanagar.

The amalgamation of the combined medical cadre took effect from 1 April 1946. It was specifically stated that the amalgamation of medical services was part of the larger policy laid down by the Government of India under which other classes of officers serving in the frontier were planned to be similarly amalgamated into one cadre.[84] Mr J.P. Mills, the Adviser to the Governor of Assam on Tribal Areas, was reportedly in the process of creating a central cadre of administrative officers for the Agency under the direct control of the Government of India. With resource inputs from the 'Post-War Five Year Plan', it was estimated that by 1951–2 the medical establishment in the Agency would increase to six AS, thirty-nine SAS, one lady doctor, forty compounders, and fourteen midwives. Mr R.W. Godfrey, the Secretary to the Governor of Assam, argued that this number was sufficient to form a separate cadre which he suggested to be named as 'North East Frontier Medical Service'.[85] It is important to note that the proposed administrative re-organization of NEFA in the wake of as well as after World War II was first experimented with medical services.

Initiatives under the 'Post-War Development Programme'

The vicissitudes of the war brought home a lesson long kept pending by the colonial authorities, viz., to bring the tribes of NEFT under direct administrative control. As soon as the war was over, a five-year plan of road improvement and construction was conceived by the Government of India and finalized at a conference of the Chief Engineers held at Nagpur. This was known as the Nagpur Plan and was subsequently termed the 'Post-War Development Programme'.[86] An offshoot of this was the 'Post-War Reconstruction Plan' devised by the Government of India under which extension of basic health services and medical infrastructure was planned for the NEFT and the Naga Hills.[87] The so-named 'Post-War Five Year Plan' was a part of this programme.

The plan spoke about 'yardsticks for future administration' of the NEFT tuned to the political and strategic necessities. Thus, under the 'yardsticks', subjects like agriculture, medicine, and education were identified as 'Nation Building Departments'. A contended loyal population, went the argument, was a strategic necessity of highest importance.[88] The expansion of administrative control in the frontier needed to be preceded and facilitated by medical services. The proposal for the expansion of healthcare measures under the plan is shown in Table 2.12.

The suggestions were accepted by the Government of India and directed to be put into effect. It was agreed to give priority to the construction of buildings required for reorganization of the medical establishment in the 'medical section' of the plan.[89] Consequently, an amount of Rs.2,50,000 was sanctioned for the reconstruction of the Base Hospital at Pasighat.[90] The hospital which was staffed and paid out of the provincial cadre and provincial funds was to be taken over by the Agency.[91] With more medical establishments in sight, literate local girls and boys began to be trained as nurses and hospital attendants but the scheme failed because of lack of qualified candidates.[92]

Table 2.12: Medical Proposals under the Five Years Post-War Reconstruction Plan for Sadiya, Tirap, and Balipara Frontier Tracts, 1946

Hospitals	
Class of Hospital	*Place*
One 35-bedded hospital	Pasighat
One 145-bedded leper colony near	Pasighat
14 A Class Hospital (17 beds including 5 females and 2 isolation)	Riga, Hayuliang, Temai, Foothills (Charduar), Rupa, Dirangdzong, Duta, H.Q. of P.O. Tirap F.T., Tuen-Sang, Pelu, Dambuk, Chowkhan, Sanpura, Along
16 B Class Hospital (8 beds)	Walong, Changuinti, Pangin, Karko, Naga Hills, Kalaktang, Jamiri, Posa, Pigeronge, Rilenka, in Tirap Frontier, in Naga Hills, Puging, Jido
Housing arrangements for staffs	In all places

	Staff		
	Required under the Present Scheme	*Already Sanctioned*	*Now Required*
1.	Assistant Surgeons - 6	4	2
2.	Sub-Assistant Surgeons - 39	14	25
3.	Lady Doctor - 1	–	1
4.	Compounders - 40	17	23
5.	Midwives - 14	–	14
6.	Cooks - 33	–	33
7.	Ward Servants - 17	–	17
8.	Sweepers - 34	–	34
9.	Peons - 37	9	28
10.	Medicine Carriers - 34	8	26
11.	Rural Health Inspectors - 3	1	2
12.	Vaccinators - 6	4	2
13.	Malaria Inspectors - 2	–	2

Financial Statement for Five Years		
Year	*Expenditure (in Rs.)*	*Remarks*
First Year: 1948–49	13,89,748	The decrease in projected expenditure in later years was due to cutting in the Non-recurring Expenditure in buildings.
Second Year: 1949–50	8,09,300	
Third Year: 1950–51	9,16,772	
Fourth Year: 1951–52	8,45,488	
Fifth Year: 1952–53	5,16,812	

Source: Niazi to the Governor, Medical Department, NEFA Branch, File No. 33/29 of 1946, SAGAP, Itanagar. Copied verbatim, abridged.

The expanded health establishment was to be organized under a hierarchical medical administration with the Civil Surgeon as the controlling officer and the respective Political Officers and Assistant Political Officers exercising administrative control over the medical staff in their jurisdiction. This was an early experiment of what later became known as 'Single Line' administration, a system where the head of civil administration exercised direct control over other departments within their jurisdiction. A set of 'standing orders' meant for medical officers were prepared under which respect to tribal customs and other professional matters were outlined (see Appendix II). Under this scheme, the doctors were expected to learn the local languages and were identified as the Political Officer's 'most useful ambassadors'.[93]

It is evident that the expanded and amalgamated medical services in the post-war period were coopted under the Post-War Reconstruction Plan. However, the objective of creating a 'North East Frontier Medical Service' could not be materialized because the Government of India was facing an entirely different political scenario at the time, namely the transfer of power. So, the Governor of Assam was asked to postpone the matter of creating a separate medical cadre for NEFT until the constitutional position of the Tribal Areas in Assam was clarified under the new Constitution (of Independent India).[94]

Thus, in the last years of the colonial period, some more dispensaries were opened, and concrete efforts were initiated to establish a unified medical administration, a process which ended with the temporarily amalgamated medical service for the North East Frontier Tract.

Within three decades, the military and political expeditions of 1912–15 were carried out, medicine entered in the lexicon of the regular policy decisions relating to the NEFT, informed by, and tuned to the strategic concerns. Medicine and healthcare administration was pushed ahead of the proposed extension of regular administration in the region. Hospitals were opened in the administrative and military headquarters located in the foothill stations like Pasighat, Sadiya, Charduar, and Lokra. Dispensaries in the hills were attached to the strategically located Assam Rifles outposts like Jamiri, Rupa, Dirangzong, Balek, Pangin, Denning, etc. Many ad hoc dispensaries were opened in the Tirap during the war. Overall, from an instrument of diplomacy, medicine acquired institutional garbs. However, this process could not be completed due to the transfer of power and the anomalous position of the NEFT in the intervening period before the Constitution of Independent India came into effect in January 1950.

Notes

1. Shiela Bora, 'American Baptist Missionaries' Ethnological Writings: The Singphos and the Namsang Nagas', in *Pre-Colonial History and Traditions of Arunachal Pradesh*, ed. Sudhir Kumar Singh and Ashan Riddi, Guwahati: DVS Publishers, 2017, pp. 314–42.
2. The abandoned mission of 1839–40 amongst the tribes of what today is Tirap was part of the Shan Mission. Frederick S. Downs, *History of Christianity in India*, vol. V, part 5, Bengaluru: The Church History Association of India, 2003, p. 78.

3. Bora, 'American Baptist', p. 339.
4. N.M. Krick, 'Account of an Expedition among the Abors in 1853', in *India's North East Frontier in the Nineteenth Century*, ed. and comp. Verrier Elwin, Bombay: Oxford University Press, 1959, pp. 236–48.
5. J. Errol Gray, 'A Tour in the Singpho Country', in *India's North East*, ed. and comp. Elwin, p. 422.
6. In 1891, only about 1.37 per cent of Christians enumerated in the census lived outside Meghalaya (Garos, Khasis, and Jaintias) and Assam (plains tribe). For details on this and the phenomenal growth of Christianity in Mizoram, Manipur, and Nagaland (with the exception of the Ao Naga, most of whom were already converted) in the first half of the twentieth century see Downs, *History of Christianity*, Ch. IV, pp. 94–137.
7. Bose, *History of Arunachal*, pp. 120, 210, 211.
8. Agnus Hamilton, *In Abor Jungles of North East India*, New Delhi: Mittal Publications, 2003, pp. 331–42.
9. Ibid., pp. 332–5.
10. Major C. Bliss to the Inspector General of Police, Assam, Foreign Department Proceedings, Secret External, November 1912, Nos. 599–690, Appendix E, 'General Remarks', p. 52, NAI, New Delhi.
11. Report by Capt. G.A. Nevill on the Aka Promenade, 1913–14, Foreign and Political Department Proceedings, Secret E, April 1915, Nos. 64–66, Part I, pp. 8,10, NAI, New Delhi.
12. Ibid., p. 8.
13. Ibid., Appendix No. 2.
14. Ibid.
15. Ibid.
16. Foreign Department Proceedings, Est. July 1913, nos. 32–3, Part B, NAI, New Delhi.
17. DC Lakhimpur to the Deputy Surgeon General, Eastern Frontier Districts, Letter. No. G-379, Shillong dated 29 May 1882, Assam Secretariat, Home (B), Medical and Sanitation, Jan/83, 21–5, ASA, Dispur.
18. Goswami, *History of Assam*, p. 151.
19. Kennedy to the Secretary to the Govt of India, Home Department, letter No. 5385M, dated 12 December 1912, File No. M.O./12 (M)

of 1914, Assam Secretariat, Municipal Department, Medical-A, March 1914, No. 3, p. 1, State Archives, Government of Arunachal Pradesh, Itanagar (SAGAP), Itanagar.

20. Worgan to Second-Secretary, File No. M.O./12 (M) of 1914, Assam Secretariat, Municipal Department, Medical-A, March 1914, Nos. 3–11, p. 1, SAGAP, Itanagar.
21. Assam Secretariat, Education Department, Medical-A, March 1924, Nos. 1–12, p. 4, SAGAP, Itanagar.
22 Kennedy to Comptroller, File No. M.O./12 (M) of 1914, Assam Secretariat, Municipal Department, Medical-A, March 1914, Nos. 3–11, p. 1, SAGAP, Itanagar.
23. Kennedy to Chief Secretary, File No. M.O./12 (M) of 1914, Assam Secretariat, Municipal Department, Medical-A, March 1914, Nos. 3–11, p. 2, SAGAP, Itanagar.
24. Notification No. 4436 M. by the Chief Commissioner of Assam, File No. M.O./12 (M) of 1914, Assam Secretariat, Municipal Department, Medical-A, March 1914, No. 3, p. 3, SAGAP, Itanagar.
25. Telegram No. 3107 dated 30 May 1913 of Civil Surgeon, NEF to the IGCH, Assam, File No. M.O./12 (M) of 1914, Assam Secretariat, Municipal Department, Medical-A, March 1914, Nos. 3–11, p. 3, SAGAP, Itanagar.
26. Kennedy to the Secretary, the Govt of India, File No. M.O./12 (M) of 1914, Assam Secretariat, Municipal Department, Medical-A, March 1914, Nos. 3–11, SAGAP, Itanagar.
27. Chief Commissioner's Tour notes on the North-East Frontier dated 28 December 1913, Assam Secretariat, Political-A, March 1914, Nos. 38–40, File No. File No. F(N)/16 of 1914, SAGAP, Itanagar.
28. S. Dutta Choudhury, ed., *Gazetteer of India: Arunachal Pradesh: East and West Sing Districts*, Itanagar: Government of Arunachal Pradesh, 1994, p. 294.
29. Governor's Secretariat, Excluded Areas Records, File No. S-132/ M of 1919, p. 3, SAGAP, Itanagar.
30. Assam Secretariat, Education Department, Medical-A, March 1924, Nos. 1–12, pp. 6–14, SAGAP, Itanagar.
31. Ibid., p. 16.
32. Reid, *History of Frontier Areas*, p. 242.

33. Ibid., pp. 242–43.
34. Civil Surgeon, Sadiya Frontier Tract to the IGCH, Assam, 25 July 1925, Assam Secretariat, Medical-A, March 1928, No. 66, p. 1, SAGAP, Itanagar. From the official correspondence, it appears that in 1914, a civil hospital, as distinct from dispensaries, which primarily catered to the military personnel and colonial officials, was formally started. Before this, the military surgeon at Sadiya catered to minor cases of injury and disease of the visiting tribesmen. Vide DC Lakhimpur to the Deputy Surgeon General, Eastern Frontier Districts, Letter. No. G-379, Shillong, dated 29 May 1882, Assam Secretariat, Home (B), Medical and Sanitation, Jan/83, 21–5, ASA, Dispur.
35. Civil Surgeon, Sadiya Frontier Tract to the IGCH, Assam 25 July 1925, Assam Secretariat, Medical-A, March 1928, No. 66, p. 2, SAGAP, Itanagar.
36. Inspection remarks of the IGCH dated 19 January 1926, Assam Secretariat, Medical-A, March 1928, No. 70, p. 3, SAGAP, Itanagar.
37. Friel to the Secretary to the Government of India, Department of Education, Health and Lands, Assam Secretariat, Medical-A, March 1928, No. 77, pp. 11–12, SAGAP, Itanagar.
38. Bajpai to the Secretary to the Government of Assam, Local Self Government Department, dated 13 April 1928, Assam Secretariat, Medical-A, June 1928, No. 84, p. 8, SAGAP, Itanagar.
39. Inspection remarks made by the Governor of Assam on the Denning Civil Dispensary on 1 February 1928, Assam Secretariat, Medical-A, June 1928, No. 83, p. 8, SAGAP, Itanagar.
40. Dundas to the Chief Secretary to the Chief Commissioner of Assam, Shillong dated Camp Pasighat, the 17 December 1918, Governor's Secretariat, Excluded Areas Records, Nos. 190–3, Municipal Dept, Sanitation Branch, File No. S-1/1919, SAGAP, Itanagar.
41. Governor's Secretariat, Excluded B, Programmes for September 1938, No. 553, p. 3, SAGAP, Itanagar; and Calvert to the Secretary to the Governor of Assam, Governor's Secretariat, Excluded B, Programmes for September 1938, No. 566, p. 19, SAGAP, Itanagar.
42. Census 1951: Assam: North East Frontier Agency District Census Handbook, p. x. For a detailed history of the premier frontier force,

see L.W. Shakespear, *History of the Assam Rifles*, 1929; rpt, Sussex, England: Naval and Military Press, 2005.

43. Assam Secretariat, Medical Department, Medical-A, June 1933, Nos. 3–5, p. 1, SAGAP, Itanagar.
44. Ibid.
45. Assam Secretariat Proceedings, Medical Department, Medical-A, June 1933, No. 3, p. 1, SAGAP, Itanagar.
46. Nevill to the Under Secretary to the Government of Assam dated Lokra 1 November 1926, Assam Secretariat, Medical-B, June 1928, Nos. 109–15, File No. PH/706, SAGAP, Itanagar.
47. S. Dutta Choudhury, ed., *Gazetteer of India: Arunachal Pradesh: East Kameng, West Kameng and Tawang Districts*, Itanagar: Government of Arunachal Pradesh, 1996, p. 243.
48. Reid, *History of Frontier Areas*, p. 291.
49. Ibid., 292.
50. Assam Secretariat Proceedings, Excluded Areas Records, Notes, Political-A, December 1929, Nos. 54–6, pp. 1–2, SAGAP, Itanagar.
51. Soames to the Secretary to the Government of India dated Shillong the 27 September 1929, Assam Secretariat Proceedings, Excluded Areas Records, Notes, Political-A, December 1929, Nos. 54–6, pp. 1–2, SAGAP, Itanagar.
52. Abridged from Soames to the Foreign Secretary to the Government of India dated 19 January 1927, Assam Secretariat, Medical-B, June 1928, Nos. 109–15, File No. PH/706, Statement II, SAGAP, Itanagar.
53. '5 Years Post War Reconstruction Plan for the Assam Tribal Areas', F/No. 33/29 of 1946/ Medical Department/ NEFA Branch, SAGAP, Itanagar.
54. Bose, *History of Arunachal*, p. 186.
55. Medical Department, NEFA Branch, File No. 6/37 of 1945 (P-II), SAGAP, Itanagar; and Political Officer to the Civil Surgeon, Letter No. Tbl.V-I/46/784 dated 26-7-46, Governor's Secretariat, File No. A.1050/46, SAGAP, Itanagar.
56. Godfrey to the Secretary to the Government of India, Letter No. 6/ Med-51/46/14-Ad. dated Shillong the 7 November 1946, Governor's Secretariat, File No. A.1050/46, SAGAP, Itanagar.

57 S. Dutta Choudhury, ed., *Gazetteer of India: Arunachal Pradesh: Tirap District*, Itanagar: Government of Arunachal Pradesh, 2008, p. 206.

58. Das to the Political Officer, U/O No. 3987 dated Sadiya the 3rd October 1945, Medical Department, NEF Branch, File No. 1/37(d) (ii) of 1945, SAGAP, Itanagar.
59. Furer-Haimendorf, *The Apatanis*, p. 2.
60. Medical Department, Medical Branch, File No. 24/20 of 1945, SAGAP, Itanagar.
61. Alan Macfarlane and Mark Turin, 'Obituary: Professor Christoph von Fürer-Haimendorf 1909–1995', *Bulletin of the School of Oriental and African Studies*, University of London, vol. 59, no. 3, 1996, p. 549.
62. Adviser to the IGCH, Assam, Memo No. Tr. 160/45/1- Ad. dated Shillong the 4th January 1946, Medical Department, North East Frontier Branch, File No. 7/6(c) of 1945, SAGAP, Itanagar.
63. Neal to the IGCH, Office of the Adviser to the Governor of Assam on Tribal Affairs, File No. A 1159 of 1947, SAGAP, Itanagar.
64. Ibid.
65. Ursula Graham Bower, *The Hidden Land: Mission to a Far Corner of India*, New York: William Morrow & Company, 1953.
66. Ibid., p. 47.
67. Medical Department, Medical Branch, File No. 24/20 of 1945, SAGAP, Itanagar.
68. There is no elaboration about the position of the Dzongpen. 'Dzong' means 'fort'. The Dzongpen must have been the ecclesiastical-cum-revenue head of the town in eastern Bhutan bordering Tawang and West Kameng district.
69. Adviser to the Governor of Assam to Niazi, Medical Department, NEFA Branch, File No. 15/29 of 1945, SAGAP, Itanagar.
70. 'Tour diary of the P.O. Sadiya for the year 1935', Assam Secretariat, Excluded Area Records, Pol-B, September 1936, Nos. 566–92, SAGAP, Itanagar.
71. Ibid.
72. Medical Department, NEFA Branch, File No. 13/29 of 1945, SAGAP, Itanagar.

73. APO, Pasighat to PO, Sadiya, Memo No. 201 SD, dated 22 June/45, Medical Department, NEFA Branch, File No. 15/29 of 1945, SAGAP, Itanagar.
74. IGCH to the Governor's Secretary, Assam Governor's Secretariat, Military Secretary's Office 1945, Notes, File No. A 1045/56, SAGAP, Itanagar.
75. Bhatia to Governor's Secretary, u/o No. 244, dated 9.1.46, Assam Governor's Secretariat, Military Secretary's Office 1945, Notes, File No. A 1045/56, SAGAP, Itanagar.
76. The term 'Agency' is commonly been used in the contemporary official records to refer to the NEFT, through it was in 1954 that the name North East Frontier Agency (NEFA) formally replaced the NEFT.
77. Walker to Secretary to the Governor of Assam, No. 3457 G. dated 24 October 1945, Medical Department, NEF Branch, File No. 1/37(d)(ii) of 1945, SAGAP, Itanagar.
78. Das to the Political Officer, U/O No. 3987 dated Sadiya 3 October 1945, Medical Department, NEF Branch, File No. 1/37(d) (ii) of 1945, SAGAP, Itanagar.
79. IGCH, Assam, U/O No. 13958/NEF dated 15 November, 1945, Medical Department, NEFA Branch, File No. 47/37-D of 1945, SAGAP, Itanagar.
80. Assam Governor's Secretariat, Military Secretary's Office, 1945, Notes, File No. A 1045/56, SAGAP, Itanagar.
81. Copied verbatim from Das to the Political Officer, U/O No. 3987, dated Sadiya 3 October 1945, Medical Department, NEF Branch, File No. 1/37(d)(ii) of 1945, SAGAP, Itanagar.
82. Saikia to the Adviser, letter No. 5354-55/MI dated 30 April 1945, File No. 47/37-D of 1945, Medical Department, NEFA Branch, SAGAP, Itanagar; and Assam Governor's Secretariat, Military Secretary's Office, 1945, File No. A 1045/56, SAGAP, Itanagar.
83. 'Minutes of meeting held in the External Affairs Department on the 22 August 1945 to consider the policy for the Tribal Areas of N.E.F.', Assam Governor's Secretariat, Military Secretary's Office, 1945, File No. A 1045/56, SAGAP, Itanagar.
84. Mills to the IGCH, Memo No. 6/Med-16/46/64-Ad., Assam Gov-

ernor's Secretariat, Military Secretary's Office, 1945, File No. A 1045/56, SAGAP, Itanagar.

85. Godfrey to the Secretary to the Government of India, Letter No. 6/ Med-16/46/81-Ad., Assam Governor's Secretariat, Military Secretary's Office, 1945, File No. A 1045/56, SAGAP, Itanagar.
86. Census of India, 1951, Volume XII: Assam, Manipur and Tripura, Part I-A, Report, p. 285.
87. GED Walker, P.O., Sadiya FT dated 20 Nov 1945 to the Adviser to Governor and Niazi to the Adviser to the Governor of Assam, dated Shillong the 11 June 1946, Medical Department, NEFA Branch, File No. 33/29 of 1946, SAGAP, Itanagar.
88. Walker to the Adviser, Medical Department, NEFA Branch, File No. 33/29 of 1946, SAGAP, Itanagar.
89. Secretary to the Adviser to the Governor of Assam for Tribal Areas and States to the IGCH, Assam, dated Shillong the 22 May 1947, Governor's Secretariat, Military Secretary's Office, File No. A 1005/47, SAGAP, Itanagar.
90. Letter No. 235/HP/1 dated 25 July 1947, Medical-B, NEFA Branch, File No. 80/6 (c) of 1947, SAGAP, Itanagar.
91. Adviser to Chief Secretary dated Shillong the 10th February, 1948, Office of the Adviser to the Governor of Assam for Tribal Areas, File No. Med/11/48, SAGAP, Itanagar.
92. Medical Department, File No. 163/14 of 1948, SAGAP, Itanagar.
93. Neal to Bhatia, Governor's Secretariat, Military Secretary's Office, File No. A 1005/47, SAGAP, Itanagar.
94. Under Secretary, External Affairs Department to the Secretary to the Governor of Assam, Memo No. F. 14(8)-E/46 dated Shimla 23 October 1946, Assam Governor's Secretariat, Military Secretary's Office, 1945, File No. A 1045/56, SAGAP, Itanagar.

3

Integrating a Virgin Frontier

Expansion of the Medical Department, 1950–1987

In the early decades of the post-Independence period, medicine emerged as the most important field of government relief and development measures. That way, the emphasis on medical, as against other means of government influence, was no different from that of the preceding period. However, its meaning and scope were much wider and more effective. This was most notably seen in the expansion of the health department during the period which, compared to other government departments of the time, was well advanced and provided with the latest medical technology available at the time.

Carrying Over from the Post-War Initiatives, 1946–51

The actual expansion of the healthcare system and standardization of medical administration in Arunachal was accomplished in the post-Independence period. During the hiatus in the government policy in the intervening period of the transfer of power and coming into effect of the Constitution of Independent India, medical administration was carried out in an ad hoc manner under the Post-War Five-Year Plan, covering the period from 1946 to 1951. The temporarily amalgamated North East Frontier Agency (NEFA) medical service formed the basic structure of medical administration. A permanent medical department was yet to emerge, but so was the general administrative set-up.

This temporary measure was continued till budgetary allocations were provided under the Five-Year Plans by the Government of Independent India. Thus, by the quarter end of 30 June 1949, the total sanctioned strength of medical staff under the Post-War Five-Year Plan in the North East Frontier Tract (NEFT) including the Tuensang Area (transferred to Nagaland in 1951) was 8 CAS (Class II), 2 compounders, 9 peons, 9 medicine carriers, and 5 vaccinators.[1] The annual report of the NEFA Medical Department on the working of the outpost and dispensaries for the year 1948 provided a summary of medical facilities, staff, prevalent diseases, and the number of patients treated which is shown in Tables 3.1 (a), (b), (c), and (d).

It can be seen in that the expansion of healthcare facilities and appointment of more medical staff under the Post-War Five-Year Plan took place after 1947. Treatment of patients in indoor units started and the number of outdoor patients increased over the years such that the percentage increase in the total number of patients treated from 1947 to 1948 alone was 37.70 per cent. Malaria was the most prevalent disease and roughly constituted one-third of the total number of patients treated in 1948.

The establishment of hospitals and dispensaries alone was not considered sufficient to attract people from interior villages to come for treatment unless the people were made aware of the benefits of modern medical treatment.[2] This reflected the growing realization in the NEFA policy circle of the need to impart awareness on health and sanitation. The 'propaganda works' in the villages, first proposed by P.C. Das, CS Sadiya, in 1945, by the touring doctors on sanitation and health continued to be emphasized. Tools of 'educative propaganda' on health and sanitation like 'magic lanterns' for use by the Mobile Health Units were distributed to the respective Political Officers at Sadiya, Pasighat, Margherita, Charduar, Kimin, and Tuensang.[3]

The various posts under the medical establishment were renewed on an annual basis with more posts created as requirements arose. Diseases like leprosy, which required special treatment, were also incorporated in this scheme with leper sana-

Table 3.1a: Dispensaries in NEFA, 1948

	Functioning			Newly Opened	
	Place/Name	*Hospital Facility*		*Place/Name*	*Facility*
1.	Hayuliang dispensary	Hospital facilities with 6 beds			
			1	Along(Aalo) dispensary in the Siang valley	Hospital facilities with 6 beds
2.	Chingwinti	ditto 7 beds			
3.	Walong	ditto 4 beds			
4.	Tezu	ditto			
5.	Khonsa	ditto 6 beds			
6.	Dilli Road Project	ditto 14 beds			
7.	Pangin dispensary	ditto 8 beds	2	But Outpost dispensary in the Sela Sub-Agency	ditto 5 beds
8.	Riga	ditto 6 beds			
9.	Itinerating dispensary, Siang valley, Pasighat	NA			
10.	Foothills dispensary	NA			
11.	Dirangdzong	Hospital facilities with 9 beds	3	Namdang Road Project Dispensary (opened in November 1948)	NA
12.	Rupa	Ditto 16 beds			
13.	Kore	Ditto 10 beds			
14.	Kimin	Ditto 6 beds			

Source: Abridged from the Medical Department, NEFA Branch, File No. 11/39 of 1949, SAGAP, Itanagar.

Table 3.1b: Strength of the Medical Staff in NEFA, 1948

	Name of Post/ Designation	*Total*	*Remarks*	*Commendable Doctors*
1.	Civil Surgeon	1	The CS was in charge of Sadiya and Tirap FT	Dr Thantluanga, AS (I) Dr S.R. Marak, AS (I) Dr Hem Kanta Baruah, AS (II) Dr Dinanath Bora, AS (II) Dr Amulya Chandra Chakrabaty, AS (II) Dr Rajendra Nath Boruah, AS (II) Dr Rajani Kanta Gogoi, AS (II)
2.	AS (Class I)	4		
3.	AS (Class II)	19	Out of sanctioned strength of 25, upto 31 December 1948	
4.	Compounders	6	The sanctioned strength of compounders was 23	
5.	Rural Health Inspectors	1		
6.	Vaccinators	7		

Source: Abridged from the Medical Department, NEFA Branch, File No. 11/39 of 1949, SAGAP, Itanagar.

Table 3.1c: Total Number of Patients Treated, 1947–48

Total Number of Patients				*Remarks*
1947		*1948*		
Indoor	Outdoor	Indoor	Outdoor	There was an increase of 17,058, i.e. 37.70 % from 1947 to 1948 in the number of patients treated. The highest number of patients treated was in the itinerating Pasighat (14,258) and the lowest was in the But Outpost Dispensary (303)
421	44,609	736	61,352	
Total=45,030		Total=62,088		

Source: Abridged from the Medical Department, NEFA Branch, File No. 11/39 of 1949, SAGAP, Itanagar.

toriums set up in places like Pasighat, Along (Aalo), and Sangti (in Dirang Dzong). Thus, when the Post-War Five-Year Plan ended in 1951, there was a substantial increase in health facilities across the NEFA. The name of doctors at the time is shown in Table 3.2 and the strength of the medical staff in Table 3.3.

Table 3.1d: Prevalent Diseases, 1948

	Name of Disease	*Number of Patients*	*Number of Patients per Hundred*	*Remarks*
1.	Dysentery	1,198	Malaria was the most prominent disease in the tribal areas; sanction of 5 malaria inspectors under consideration of the government and anti-malarial measures to be taken up when the posts were sanctioned, trained Malaria Inspectors already appointed. Experimental treatment with iodized salt started for treating goitre. 2.20 3.50 33.09 4.09	
2.	Diarrhoea	1,923		
3.	Malaria	18,179		
4.	Diseases of the eye	2,252		

contd.

	Name of Disease	Number of Patients	Number of Patients per Hundred	Remarks
5.	Scabies	4,481	8.14	Other diseases
6.	Goitre	5,410	9.84	Leprosy: prevalent; a leper colony under construction in Abor (Adi) Hills near Pasighat.
7.	Diseases of bones, joints, muscles, etc.	3,274	5.95	Cholera: Nil Smallpox: 2 cases
8.	Ulcerative inflammation	4,551	8.28	Kala Kala Azar: 2 cases; 1 in Subansiri Area and 1 in Mishmi Hills
9.	Other disease of the skin, nail, etc.	2,050	3.73	Measles: there was an epidemic of measles in Siang valley and 622 cases were treated in all.
10.	Injuries, general and local	3,045	5.54	Venereal diseases: 356 cases of syphilis and 127 cases of gonococcal infection treated during the year. Out of 356 cases of syphilis, 317 cases were treated in Abor (Adi) Hills alone.
11.	Diseases of the respiratory system	5,305	9.65	Buildings
12.	Diseases of the stomach	1,721	3.13	There was no permanent building in the agency. Most of the dispensary buildings and staff quarters were of kutcha type.
13.	Other diseases of the digestive system	1,545	2.81	
14.	Total	54,934	100	

Source: Abridged from the Medical Department, NEFA Branch, File No. 11/39 of 1949, SAGAP, Itanagar.

Table 3.2: Strength of Civil Assistant Surgeons (Class II) in NEFA, 1951

	Name of Outpost Dispensary	*Name of Doctor*
Naga Hills	Tuensang	Dr Lalthanliana
Sela Sub-agency	But	Dr Narendra Nath Boorah (yet to join)
	Rupa	Dr Rebati Mohan Bora
	Dirangdzong	Dr Kamaniya Kar
	Foothills	Dr Nalin Chandra Barua (yet to join)
	Leave reserve	Dr Basanta Kumar Pathak (yet to join)
Subansiri	Kimin	Dr Aurobindo Paul
	Sagalee	Dr S. Kalita
	Ziro	Dr N.C. Das
	Itinerating, Subansiri	Dr Nikunja Behari Das (yet to join)
Siang valley	Aalo	Dr Amalananda Roy
	Panging (Pangin)	Dr Sumilan Bhadra
	Daring (Dari)	Dr A.C. Chakravarty
		Dr S.N. Ghosh (on leave)
	Riga	Dr Kushadhar Saikia
	Itinerating	Dr Prabuddha Nath Bhattacharjee
	Gunjeng Leprosy Colony	Dr Subodh Chandra Bhattacharjee
Lohit valley	Tezu	Dr Dinanath Bora
Mishmi Hills	Dambuk	Dr Umanath Bhuyan
	Nizamghat	Dr Nizamuddin Ahmad
	Hayuliang	Dr Prafulla Chandra Barua
	Changwinti	Dr Bimala Charan Dhar
	Walong	Dr Mahendra Ch. Goswami (on leave)
	Itinerating	Dr Panchu Gopal Dey (yet to join)
Tirap Frontier Tract	Khonsa	Dr Jalauddin Borbora
	Namdang Road Project	Dr Dwijendra Lal Roy
	Itinerating for Tirap FT	Dr Paresh Chandra Sarkar (yet to join)
	Forest Dispensary Tirap	Dr Veronica Nui Hmar
	Chowkham	Vacant

Source: Copied verbatim from Personal Assistant to the IGCH, Assam to the Secretary to the Governor of Assam dated 8/1/51, File No. Med/19/49, Medical Department, NEFA, SAGAP, Itanagar.

Table 3.3: Strength of the Medical Staff in NEFA, 1951

Name of Post	*No. of Sanctioned Posts*
Civil Assistant Surgeon (I)	6
Civil Assistant Surgeon (II)	34
Compounder	27
Dresser	4
Rural Health Inspector	3
Vaccinator	15
Senior Malaria Inspector	1
Malaria Inspector	3
Malaria Sub-Inspector	5
Insect Collector	3
Mechanic	1
Head Assistant (Office of the Civil Surgeon)	1
Accountant	1
Upper Division Assistant(in the office of the IGCH, Assam)	1
Upper Division Assistant	4
Lower Division Assistant	11
Peon, Orderly, Medical Attendant, Medicine Carrier, Chowkidar	71
Interpreter	3
Sweepers	10
Total number of sanctioned posts	204

Source: Medical Department, NEFA, File No. 11/39 of 1951, SAGAP, Itanagar.

The Japanese invasion in the North-East during World War II has been credited with bringing infrastructure projects like civil airlines, major road projects, etc., to north-east India.[4] It may also be argued that the War was a blessing in disguise for NEFA in so far as it pushed medical facilities ahead of administrative reorganization of the region. The reforms and expansions undertaken during the post-War period provided a framework upon which the medical department of NEFA, generously cushioned by the national Five-Year Plans, was subsequently shaped.

Formation of the NEFA Medical Department and Growth under Five-Year Plans

It was also considered important that the office of the nodal medical officer, the Civil Surgeon, was established nearer to the villages in order to develop closer ties with the people and for generating a better understanding of the actual medical situation. The first effort in this direction was made when the office of the Civil Surgeon was transferred from Shillong to Pasighat with effect from 15 November 1949 'in the interest of public service'.[5]

The move to bring public welfare measures, of which medical was the most important one, nearer to the people was further strengthened when the NEFA Medical Department was formed in 1951.[6] In the same year, the designation of the Civil Surgeon was changed to Chief Medical Officer (CMO) who was placed in the rank of a Lieutenant Colonel.[7] Since February 1955, the NEFA Medical Department began to be headed by the Director of Health Services (DHS) under the general guidance of the NEFA administration. The list of the Civil Surgeons and Director of Health Services are given in Appendices IV and V.

The promulgation of the North-East Frontier Area (Administration) Regulation, 1954 formally gave a distinct administrative identity to the frontier. As intended, this facilitated exclusive focus of the government on the frontier and the same was reflected in the separate budgetary allocations of the successive Five-Year Plans, and in the increasing number of health facilities being opened, as shown in Tables 3.4 to 3.8.

Right from the First Plan, 'medical' formed an important component of the budgetary allocations for the NEFA; till the Third Plan, it constituted an independent budgetary sub-head. From the Fifth Plan, medical was put under 'social service' as more development sub-heads were created. This did not suggest a decline in the importance of health in the budgetary provisions but reflected the holistic scope development planning in NEFA began

Table 3.4: Priorities of the First Three Five-Year Plans for NEFA Compared (figures in brackets indicate the plan outlay in rupees lakh)

Priority Assigned in Each Plan	*First Five-Year Plan (1951–6)*		*Second Five-Year Plan (1956–7 to 1960–1)*		*Third Five-Year Plan (1961–2 to 1965–6)*	
	Name of the Development Heads	*Per cent of Allotment of the Outlay*	*Name of the Development Heads*	*Per cent of Allotment of the Outlay*	*Name of the Development Heads*	*Per cent of Allotment of the Outlay*
1	*2*	*3*	*4*	*5*	*6*	*7*
1.	Engineering	45.00 (135.00)	Engineering	37.58 (191.50)	Engineering	37.38 (265.00)
2.	Medical	21.67 (65.00)	Agriculture	22.37 (114.07)	Agriculture & CD/N.E.S.	22.08 (156.58)
3.	Education	13.94 (41.81)	Medical	15.78 (80.42)	Medical	18.76 (133.00)
4.	Agriculture	10.67 (32.00)	Education	9.81 (50.00)	Education	11.62 (82.37)
5.	Others	8.72 (26.19)	Others	14.46 (73.46)	Others	10.16 (72.05)
6.	Total	300.00		509.56		715.00

Source: Statistical Outline of North East Frontier Agency, April 1961, Shillong: Statistical Branch, NEFA, p. 29.

Table 3.5: Hospital, Dispensaries and Patients Treated, 1951–7

Sl. No.	*Year*	*Division*	*Hospitals*	*Dispensary*	*MHU*	*Total*	*Total Patients Treated*	
							Indoor	*Outdoor*
0	*1*	*2*	*3*	*4*	*5*	*6*	*7*	*8*
1.	1951	Kameng	4	4	2	10	776	15,916
		Subansiri	3	-	-	3	329	16,451
		Siang	1	9	1	11	456	46,436
		Lohit	2	6	1	9	591	31,433
		Tirap	-	4	2	6	-	15,688
		Total	10	23	6	39	2,152	1,25,924
2.	1952	Kameng	4	5	1	10	965	17,703
		Subansiri	3	4	-	7	194	12,549
		Siang	1	9	1	11	1,158	55,486
		Lohit	2	8	1	11	683	27,109
		Tirap	1	10	2	12	144	30,138
		Total	11	36	5	52	3,144	1,42,985
3.	1953	Kameng	5	6	7	18	1,019	30,332
		Subansiri	3	5	2	10	223	20,644
		Siang	2	10	6	18	1,052	47,757

contd.

Sl. No.	*Year*	*Division*	*Hospitals*	*Dispensary*	*MHU*	*Total*	*Total Patients Treated*	
							Indoor	*Outdoor*
		Tirap	1	11	4	16	301	54,480
		Total	13	40	23	76	3,314	1,83,688
4.	1954	Kameng	5	6	5	16	1,019	38,725
		Subansiri	3	3	1	7	388	37,719
		Siang	5	10	6	21	1,203	53,821
		Lohit	2	8	3	13	637	28,899
		Tirap	2	8	2	12	291	52,627
		Total	17	35	17	69	3,538	2,11,791
5.	1955	Kameng	7	4	2	13	1,192	42,622
		Subansiri	3	4	1	8	415	40,104
		Siang	2	11	1	14	1,145	67,713
		Lohit	4	6	3	13	1,010	27,053
		Tirap	2	10	3	15	273	57,769
		Total	18	35	10	63	4,035	2,35,261
6.	1956	Kameng	7	5	2	14	NA	NA
		Subansiri	3	6	1	10	NA	NA
		Siang	2	10	1	13	NA	NA

contd.

Sl. No.	*Year*	*Division*	*Hospitals*	*Dispensary*	*MHU*	*Total*	*Total Patients Treated*	
							Indoor	*Outdoor*
		Tirap	2	12	3	17	NA	NA
		Total	18	39	9	66	NA	NA
7.	1957	Kameng	7	5	2	14	NA	NA
		Subansiri	3	7	1	11	NA	NA
		Siang	2	14	1	17	NA	NA
		Lohit	4	6	2	12	NA	NA
		Tirap	2	12	3	17	NA	NA
		Total	10	44	9	71	NA	NA

Source: Statistical Outline of North East Frontier Agency: April 1958, Shillong: Statistical Branch, NEFA, p. 15.

Table 3.6: Priorities of the Fourth Five-Year Plan, 1966–71
(in rupees lakh)

Sl. No.	*Head of Development*	*Total Plan Provision*	*Per Cent of Allotment of the Outlay*
1.	Engineering	495.59	
2.	Agriculture	264.00	
3.	Forest	175.54	
4.	CD and NES	149.98	
5.	Medical and Public Health	383.66	19.25
6.	Education	317.62	
7.	Industries	54.32	
8.	Research	6.67	
9.	Publicity	41.80	
10.	Cooperation	92.67	
11.	Statistics	8.86	
12.	Strengthening of Administrative Machinery	2.00	
	Total	1,992.71	

Source: Abridged from *Statistical Outline of North East Frontier Agency, April 1966*, Shillong Statistical Department, NEFA, p. 22.

to acquire. There is a progressive increase in the budgetary allocations with two distinct phases where we notice quantum jumps—the Fourth and Sixth Plans. By the end of the Sixth Five-Year Plan (1984–5) healthcare facilities in the state included 146 allopathic, 16 homoeopathic, and 1 ayurvedic hospital with 2,013 beds, 184 doctors, and 216 nurses.[9] By 1988, this figure rose to 218 allopathic, 27 homoeopathic, and 1 ayurvedic hospital.[10] Thus, by the late 1980s, healthcare facilities penetrated most parts of the state across all administrative divisions. The tremendous expansion of healthcare facilities across the length and breadth of the frontier in the successive decades after 1950 is given in Appendices VI and VII.

Table 3.7: Sectoral Plan Outlays Since the Fifth Five-Year Plan
(in percentage)

Plan Period	*Agriculture and Allied*	*Industry and Mining*	*Power and Irrigation*	*Transport and Comm.*	*Social and Community Service*	*Economic Service*	*General Service*
V Plan	26.77	2.05	6.87	33.03	30.84	0.44	-
VI Plan	24.22	4.84	12.82	26.46	30.95	0.35	0.36
VII Plan	21.66	2.41	15.92	32.19	26.62	0.66	0.54
VIII Plan	11.26	2.82	20.59	32.13	28.77	1.28	3.15
IX Plan	13.16	1.29	20.93	26.04	33.03	3.26	2.29
X Plan	18.11	1.78	18.55	25.1	29.83	4.64	1.99

Source: Arunachal Pradesh Human Development Report, 2005, Itanagar: Department of Planning, Government of Arunachal Pradesh, 2006, p. 278.

Table 3.8: Five-Year Plans: Outlay and Expenditure (in rupees crore)

Sl. No.	*Plans*	*Period*	*Outlay*	*Expenditure*
0	*1*	*2*	*3*	*4*
1.	First Plan	1951–6	3.00	2.0122
2.	Second Plan	1956–61	5.09	3.5664
3.	Third Plan	1961–6	7.15	9.2037
4.	Annual Plan	1966–9	8.47	8.3090
5.	Fourth Plan	1969–74	17.99	21.5792
6.	Fifth Plan	1974–9	63.30	60.8628
7.	Annual Plan	1979–80	46.81	23.4100
8.	Sixth Plan	1980–5	222.90	205.8522
9.	Seventh Plan	1985–90	549.00	550.4900
10.	Annual Plan	1990–2	418.00	395.8100
11.	Eighth Plan	1992–7	1155.00	—

Source: Statistical Atlas of Arunachal Pradesh, 1995, Itanagar: Directorate of Economics and Statistics, Government of Arunachal Pradesh, p. 54.

Census, Statistical Data, and Demography

With the establishment of administrative centres and planned development programmes, statistical data on demography and other economic indicators became important exercises which in turn helped healthcare planning. The first census was carried out in NEFA as part of Assam in 1951; from 1961, it was censused separately.[11] In 1957, the NEFA Statistical Department tried to enumerate the population of the frontier and projected a population of only three lakhs. This was far below the estimate of six to eight lakhs made by the administration earlier.[12] The population enumerated in the first independent census of NEFA is shown in Table 3.9.

Increasing population contact and urbanization are considered important elements in mapping healthcare history. Apart from the environmental context, anthropologists generally include social patterns which affect health, viz., food distribution, sexual practices, hygiene, population contact, urbanization, etc.[13] From the

Table 3.9: Distribution of Population in NEFA, 1961

Sl. No.	*Name of Area/District/ Sub-Division*	*No. of Villages*	*Popula-tion*	*Population per village*	*Density (per sq. km.)*
(0)	*(1)*	*(2)*	*(3)*	*(4)*	*(5)*
	North East Frontier Agency	2,451	3,36,558	137	4.1
1.	Kameng Frontier Division	333	69,913	210	4.9
2.	Subansiri Frontier Division	583	62,090	107	5.3
3.	Siang Frontier Division	682	108,914	160	4.2
	Daporizo Sub-Division	290	24,481	84	NA
	Along Sub-Division	273	47,995	176	NA
	Pasighat Sub-Division	119	36,438	306	NA
4.	Lohit Frontier Division	604	36,050	60	1.5
	Roing Sub-Division	192	10,251	53	NA
	Tezu Sub-Division	412	25,799	63	NA
5.	Tirap Frontier Division	249	59,591	239	8.43

Source: Census of India, 1961, vol. XXIV: North East Frontier Agency, Part II-A, General Population Tables and NEFA Special Tables 5, p. 7.

historical point of view, population contact in Arunachal happened in three different ways, viz., within a particular group or community; between (some) of the communities; and, between some of the communities and the world outside. Because of difficult geographical conditions, contact within and between communities was very limited and this kept 'the people divided and short of what they needed'.[14] Intercourse with the world outside happened from three different directions: Bhutan in the west and Tibet in the north, Myanmar in the east, and Assam in the south.

Traditional migration patterns, trade routes, and political relations with the respective rulers of the Brahmaputra valley influenced the nature of population contact. Examples of the indigenous population who experienced de-population due to contact with outsiders and the resultant epidemics have been documented as in the case of the Aleuts of North America.[15]

Despite the reported cases of 'sickness carrying' (discussed in the second part of Chapter 4) and import of disease from the plains, even suggestive ideas in this regard are obfuscated by lack of empirical data on population exchange in the decades before the 1950s.

Given this shortcoming, urbanization as another reference in writing a health history is also difficult. Recent research on urbanization and the rise of mental diseases amongst the Apatanis of Ziro valley found that the indigenous belief system of 'spirit-possession' is construed as schizophrenia by modern psychiatry.[16] A thickly populated plateau and the administrative centre of the Subansiri region since the mid-1940s, Ziro experienced urbanization and professional mobility in a matter of few decades. This rapid change is cited to be the reason behind the prevalence of more mental disorders among the Apatanis than any other community in the state.[17] The study substantiates its finding by taking the example of Reru village, considered the most 'advanced'—having the highest literacy rate; producing more professionals, politicians, and businessmen; having a number of modified modern houses compared to other villages in the plateau—but with the most psychiatric cases.[18] No similar study on other regions of the state exists making the Ziro case, of one study, an inadequate sample to throw light on this aspect with respect to the whole state. Table 3.10 shows the overall population growth in the state from 1961 to 1991.

Diseases and Special Measures: Growth of Preventive Medicine

The nature of diseases recorded during the post-1950 phase was no different from those mentioned in the colonial records. The major diseases reported were respiratory disorders, diarrhoea and dysentery, skin diseases, stomach and intestinal diseases, goitre, malaria, tuberculosis, syphilis, leprosy, and others.[19] The threat of malaria,

Table 3.10: Population growth in Arunachal Pradesh, 1961–91

Year	*Size of Population*	*Growth of Population (% per annum)*	*Total ST*	*General*	*Total ST*	*General*
1961	3,36,558	2,99,944	36,614	–	–	–
1971	4,67,511	3,69,408	98,103	3.89	2.32	16.79
1981	6,31,839	4,41,167	1,90,672	3.51	1.94	9.44
1991	8,64,558	5,50,351	3,14,207	3.68	2.47	6.48

Source: Arunachal Human Development Report, 2005, Itanagar: Department of Planning, Government of Arunachal Pradesh, 2006, p. 13.

which had attracted special anti-malarial measures in the foothills of Arunachal since the 1920s, was finally brought under control. About 39.36 per cent of the patients treated in 1951 suffered from malaria and by 1963, this figure came down to 0.58 per cent.[20] The menace of malaria was controlled within the first two Five-Year Plans. This was the result of dedicated anti-malaria drives initiated by the government. For example, in 1955, 27 anti-malaria units were put into service in about 220 villages with a total population of approximately 57,000.[21] Thus, malaria was the first major disease to be brought under control in Arunachal Pradesh.

Skin diseases, tuberculosis, smallpox, and venereal diseases were the other topical diseases which attracted special attention. Skin disease, which was reported to be more prevalent in northern and north-west Siang, was correctly diagnosed in 1957 and treatment was started thereafter.[22] About 50 per cent of the people of the state were believed to have been suffering from endemic goitre during this time.[23] Iodized salts were supplied to affected areas in substantial quantities every month. Efforts were also made by the health department to know the indigenous names of goitre, iodine, and salt.[24] This was done to make public education on goitre-prevention and healthcare locally relevant by using local names in the goitre-control programmes. Popular appeal and cultural relevance were considered important to make healthcare measures effective and successful.

Latest advancements in medical technology and preventive healthcare were made use of. This is witnessed in the various vaccination programmes that were carried out as soon as they were started in the country. The Bacillus Calmette-Guérin (BCG) vaccination programme against tuberculosis was started in February 1957, the same time it was launched in the country. In two years' time, about 30,000 people were tested and 8,034 vaccinated against the disease.[25] Special officers were posted in the Health Directorate in Shillong; two of these were dedicated to malaria and smallpox respectively. In 1962, the National Smallpox Eradication Programme (NSEP) was started in the state,[26] the same year that the programme was launched in India, and four years after the World Health Organization (WHO) resolved to eradicate it globally.[27]

As part of this evolving preventive healthcare orientation of the NEFA health department, many other measures were also adopted in 1963–4: distribution of milk powder in schools through school health service; launching of mobile X-ray units; ambulance service; mobile eye teams; and mobile dental tests. The first mobile X-ray unit was proposed for Kameng Frontier Division in 1962–3 which was delayed because of Chinese aggression.[28]

Broadening the Meaning of Healthcare: Water Supply and Communication

From the Third Plan, water supply was made an integral part of the healthcare scheme.[29] Providing water supply in NEFA faced a peculiar problem—most villages were not uniformly located and in many places, they were situated far away from the source of water. The scarcity of water in many villages impeded the use of water for personal hygiene and cleanliness. The provision of tap-water supply to villages thus brought a revolutionary change in the daily hygiene of the people.

Like water supply, road connectivity was integral to the effective implementation of healthcare measures in a geographically vast and topographically challenging region. In 1947, there were only three 'jeepable' roads: Pasighat-Kobo (22 mi.) in Siang valley; Sadiya-Tezu-Denning (48 mi.) in the Lohit valley; and Stillwell Road (35 mi.) in Tirap.[30] The road network as it existed in the mid-1950s is shown in tables 3.11 (a) and (b).

Road connectivity in the early decades after the establishment of the Medical Department was negligible. In the entire Subansiri Division, there was only one porter track (Doimukh to Sagalee) leading to any interior outpost while some outposts in the foothill areas were connected to neighbouring towns in Assam by motorable roads. In the Siang Frontier Division, the situation was relatively better. Some villages near the administrative headquarters at Pasighat and Along were connected either by motorable road or mule paths. Pasighat was connected to Dibrugarh and Sadiya by waterways since the Abor Expedition (1911–12). Road connectivity in other parts of the state was fundamentally not different from the above, indicating that expansion of the healthcare system faced the problem of connectivity and transportation in the early decades after the 1950s.

Taking the Environment and Culture Along

The climatic, ecological, and geographical condition of Arunachal is a subject of many colonial and ethnological records during the nineteenth and the first half of the twentieth century. But the focus of such enquiries in the light of health and general welfare emerged only in the second half of the twentieth century under the architect of NEFA, Verrier Elwin. Elwin generated a focus on housing, dress, opium use, and food habits, etc., as important determinants in the successful implementation of healthcare measures.[31] Subse-

Table 3.11a: Jeep Roads and Mule Paths in Siang Frontier Division, 1958

	Muleable	*Motorable*	*Remarks*
Pasighat to Along	15 mi.	10 mi.	
Pasighat to Sivokorong	-	3	
Pasighat to Ledum-Tene-Rotte	8	20	
Pasighat to Oyram Ghat	-	22	Improvement in progress
Approach to Pasighat	-	-	Two miles under construction
Pasighat Town Access Road	-	6	
Balek Approach Road	-	1	
Ledum Approach Road	-	1	
Mirem Approach Road	-	1	
Ralung Rani Road	-	6	
Mirem Mikong Road	-	4	
Along Station Road	-	4	
Along to Majherbari	90	-	Under construction
Oyan Jonai Road	-	-	
Along to Pangin	20	-	
Along to Kombong	-	6	
Along to Basar OP	35	20	Only 6 miles jeepable for want of bridges
Along to Yomcha	34	-	

Source: Tables 3.11(a) and (b) extracted from 'Tour Dairy of Shri R.K. Haranga, Secretary, Supply and Transport', File No. R.46/58, NEFA Administration, Shillong, 1958, SAGAP, Itanagar.

quent studies highlighted the absence of the concept of cleanliness, paucity of clothes, distant source of water from villages, absence of windows in houses, and the resultant problem of smoke, lack of lavatory, and the custom of using the attached pigsty at the backyard in its place, etc., as important environmental factors affecting hygiene.[32] The following description of the ecological impact on the general health of the people is a representative example:

Table 3.11b: Jeep Roads and Mule Paths in Subansiri Frontier Division, 1959

	Muleable	*Motorable*	*Remarks*
Kimin to Doimukh	-	36 mi.	Motorable for all types of vehicles
Kimin to N/ Lakhimpur	-	16	Ditto
Doimukh to Drupang (via Harmutty)	-	6	Ditto
Doimukh to Drupang (via Narayanpur)	-	36	Ditto
Doimukh to Panbari (via Harmutty)	-	6	Ditto
Doimukh to Panbari (via Bihpuria)	-	31	Ditto
Doimukh to 'Daflagarh'	-	18	Ditto
Kimin to Lilabari	-	19	Ditto
Kimin to Ziro	-	57	The road made through but not yet completed 36 mi. porter tracks
Doimukh to Sagalee	-	-	

Source: Extracted from the 'Tour Dairy of Shri R.K. Haranga, Secretary, Supply and Transport', File No. R.46/58, NEFA Administration, Shillong, 1958, SAGAP, Itanagar

The climate in most parts of NEFA is rigorous, the level of living low, the standards of hygiene primitive and medical facilities scarce. As a result the mortality rate is high, particularly among children. It is only the toughest among the progeny that survive and reach adulthood. The general appearance of good health compared with the other people in the country is somewhat misleading, because it is only the best element in the population that survives. Statistical info is not available but it appears that the population among the tribals is increasing, if at all, at a very low rate.[33]

Prevalence of diseases was linked to climatic conditions: pulmonary diseases were common in the drier regions in the west and the north while goitre in the higher Himalayan ranges, and skin and stomach disorders in the wetter regions.[34] One-third of the population living below 5,000 feet was considered prone to malaria. The prolonged period of low health conditions and appearance of people as less healthy in these areas was conjectured as resulting from the general environment.

Shifting cultivation impeded the Malaria Eradication Programme because the practice made families and villages migratory; the problem of flies, mosquitoes, and other pests, such as dim-dam fly and leeches added to the general danger posed by the environment to health. Even daily habits of the people which affected health and hygiene became a matter of government health policy as reflected in these lines:

> A central fire-place in this damp and cold region is a most welcome and attractive thing, but it has a hypnosis. It does not allow people to move away easily form it. Thus, through centuries a habit has developed in these people to spit where they like and as they like. Lung diseases are consequently common among them. This is a very great problem both to the Tuberculosis worker and the health educator.[35]

Venereal diseases (VD) were reported from regions where the village community was settled and had a higher density of population, viz., the Tawang area (as reported by Kennedy earlier)[36] and the Siang region. In 1947–8 alone, about 500 cases of VD were detected and treated in the Siang region.[37] Cases were also reported from the Noklak area of Tuensang in Tirap. The idea that the communal bachelors' barrack, common to both the Siang and Tirap communities, and the assumed promiscuity prevalent in these traditional youth dormitories as the probable cause of the VDs was rejected.[38] A possible relationship between the existence of such dormitories and the spread of the VD was earlier suggested by a Political Officer.[39] Since no systemic study on the disease has been carried out in the state as, for example, in the case of the Hulis of Papua New Guinea,[40] the mere passing attention a particular social institution attracted with regard to a disease indicates the growing interest of public epidemiology of the new healthcare regime as well as the potentiality of modern medicine in the portrayal and redefining of indigenous institutions.

Military and Medicine: The Continued Relevance of the Assam Rifles Outposts

What the lack of road connectivity impeded, the presence of Assam Rifles outposts facilitated. During the pre-1950 phase, a few dispensaries attached to the military were set up in remote corners of the frontier. As seen in the previous chapter, such dispensaries were not a chance extension of the Assam Rifles outposts or road projects. These were tactfully camouflaged—goodwill-powerhouses stacked with medicines and ambassador-doctors set to project the military, the symbol of colonial power and authority, in benevolent disguise before the ever-suspicious tribes.

As a result, instead of seeing the military outposts as symbols of colonial intrusion in their area, people gratefully regarded them as a means to get medicine and relief from diseases. It is no coincidence that unlike in the nineteenth century, no major confrontation between any of the tribes and the colonial authorities took place in the first half of the twentieth century, from 1915 to 1947–50. No wonder then, it was reported that the Assam Rifles personnel shared good relationships with the people wherever they were stationed.[41] By the end of World War II, the Assam Rifles posts were located in the places as shown in Table 3.12.

In 1951–2, the strength of outposts was increased in the Sela Sub-Agency when three new outposts were established in But, Tawang, and Leyak and check-posts were established at Sangezong, Jang, Lumla, Chutangmu, and Bumla.[42] In Subansiri, outposts were opened at Ziro, Daporijo, Sagalee, Gocham, Nyapin, Kimin, and Doimukh.[43] Most of these outposts were opened to facilitate administrative reach which was happening for the first

Table 3.12: Assam Rifles Outposts in NEFT, 1946

Se La Area	Dirangdzong	½ platoon from the beginning of the year to the 2nd April 1946, 1 platoon thereafter to the end of the year	Permanent
	Rupa	1 platoon	Ditto
Siang valley Sub-Agency	Pangin	½ platoon	Ditto
	Riga	½ platoon from July 1945 to November 1945, and 1 platoon thereafter.	Ditto
	Karko	Ditto	Ditto
Lohit valley Sub-Agency	Hayuliang	½ platoon from the beginning of the year till February 1946, and 1 platoon thereafter	Ditto
	Walong (with a subsidiary post at Changwinti)	1 platoon	Ditto
Tirap Frontier Tract	Khonsa	½ platoon	Temporary

Source: J.P. Mills, Adviser to the Governor of Assam for Tribal Areas, 'Report on the Assam Tribal Areas for the year ending June 30th, 1946', Appendix II, SAGAP, Itanagar.

time in these areas. All outposts except Kimin and Doimukh were rationed through airlifting and airdropping. Malarial units were posted in all the outposts except Daporijo.

Exploring Alternative Medicine: Ayurveda and Homeopathy

The potential of herbal medicine in NEFA was recognized from an early stage; it was also expected to supplement the lack of doctors. A decision was taken to introduce alternative medicine after experience gained in such projects from Assam was consulted. Thus, in 1951, the Ayurvedic system of medicine was introduced in NEFA with the following objectives:

In view of the acute dearth of doctors willing to serve in the NEFA, the suggestion has been made that the Ayurvedic system of medicine might be introduced with advantage in our tribal areas.... It is not our intention to substitute allopathic treatment by [the]Ayurveda system of treatment in the tribal areas ... our tribal areas are rich in indigenous ingredients which are used in [the] ayurvedic system of treatment, it is desirable, as an experimental measure, to establish Ayurvedic dispensaries in two thickly populated districts of the Agency. This will also solve the problem of rendering medical aid to the tribal people, especially in the areas where there are no doctors and compounders.[44]

On 8 February 1951, three posts of Ayurvedic doctors were sanctioned in the scale pay of Civil Assistant Surgeon II.[45] They were posted at Basar in Siang, Pinziang in Tirap, and Jamiri in Kameng with one peon and one medicine carrier each. In the subsequent decades, homeopathic medicine was also introduced.

Medical Education: Nursing, Compoundry and MBBS

With the expansion of the medical department and acute shortage of candidates ready to serve in the remote areas of the frontier, it was considered important to train local youths educated in the medical profession. The first step in this direction was taken in April 1951 when six boys and three girls were admitted to compoundry and nursing courses in the Berry White Medical School at Dibrugarh (now renamed the Assam Medical College).[46] From 1950 to 1951, students were nominated for full-term medicine courses in MBBS and compoundry with a scholarship at the rate of Rs.40 per month.

Under this scheme, candidates from other tribal areas of the hills of Assam were given preference before seats were offered to plain tribes of Assam or other communities from the plains.[47] After completion of studies, the graduates were obliged to serve anywhere in NEFA for a minimum period of five years as per the scholarship bond. Within three decades, this system of medical education evolved into an important area of technical education sponsored by the state government. The total number of scholarships for the years 1986–8 is shown in Table 3.13.

Life of Medical Professionals: Infrastructure and Popular Perceptions

The spread of both the curative and preventive dimensions of healthcare meant more engagement of health professionals with people in interior areas. Despite the relative improvement in infrastructure, the medical staff continued to face many difficulties which had earlier attracted reforms in the post-War years' plan: lack of means of transportation and communication; challenging

Table 3.13: Scholarship for Medical Education, 1986–8

Year/Nominee	*Number of Students sponsored for*				
	MBBS	*Dental Surgery*	*B.Pharma*	*Nursing*	*Total*
1	*2*	*3*	*4*	*5*	*6*
1986–7	27	7	-	17	51
A.P. Tribal	22	6	-	5	33
Others	5	1	-	12	18
1987–8	32	5	1	17	55
A.P. Tribal	27	1	1	5	34
Others	5	4	-	12	21

Source: Economic Review of Arunachal Pradesh 1988, Shillong: Directorate of Economics and Statistics, Government of Arunachal Pradesh, p. 71.

topography; harsh climate; dismal conditions of hospital and dispensaries; lack of housing for staffs; diseases; and problems in pursuing people to get vaccinated, etc. Doctors had to tour the interior villages for a period ranging from 40 to 115 days a year.[48]

The memoirs of former NEFA officials like Rustomji, Kaul, Bhattacharjee, Bordoloi, Haldipur, Krishnatry, and others highlight the human and logistics challenges encountered by the healthcare workers, as also by others working in the government.[49] Some developed liking for local women, many of whom preferred to marry a government man than to be bound in abusive and, often, forlorn (because of child-) marriages, and had to be secretly hurried away to safety by the authorities in order to avoid unwanted fallouts; many others got along with the zestful tribal life, married local girls, and happily served in the hills throughout their career re-incarnating themselves as a default crusader, as well as an example of the hills-plains symbiosis in the process.

When Roing was made the headquarters of the Mishmi Hills District in May 1952, the Chidu Dispensary was shifted to Roing which, with an average of twenty-five patients per day, provided both indoor and outdoor health facilities. There was no road connectivity to Roing for the first six months after it was made the headquarters of the Mishmi Hills District.[50] At Chowkham in the Khampti area, the doctor had no residential quarters and thus had taken shelter in one of the rooms of the hospital which itself was under constant threat of flood.

In Seppa in Kameng, the hospital building was not well planned: there was no operation room, isolation rooms, dressing materials, hospital clothes, and residential quarters.[51] The hospital at Hapoli in Ziro suffered from similar problems and the habit of indiscriminate spitting by the locals added to the problem of sanitation in the hospital premises.[52] The delay in receipt of salaries for up to four to five months made the life of medical staff miserable.[53] Similar problems were reported from Sarli in Subansiri and also from Khonsa, Changlang, and Nampong in Tirap. In Sarli, the health unit was unable to cope with the rising demand because health workers sometimes proceeded on leave for prolonged period without relievers.[54] The Bhalukpong dispensary in Kameng was reportedly crowded with indoor and outdoor patients beyond its capacity even when the hospital barracks were dirty and congested.[55] The expensive laboratory equipment and X-ray machine in Pasighat hospital were not used because of the non-availability of electricity.[56]

The infrastructural challenges to healthcare delivery were compounded by some social factors. Patients cured of tuberculosis and Hansen's disease (HD or leprosy) faced social stigma, an issue elaborated in the next chapter. The response of the people to the new healthcare measures was different from place to place. At Sille in Siang, people refused to get vaccinated for reasons the healthcare workers and the administration failed to ascertain.[57] Similarly, the Nocte and the Wancho villages in Tirap were reluctant to divulge the correct names of the members of their family during the National Smallpox Eradication Programme.[58] These incidents were probably a case of initial apprehension; in 1951, people are reported to have welcomed the vaccinators during the smallpox mass vaccination against an ongoing epidemic.[59] The earlier fear of vaccination and injection was gradually discarded by the people themselves.[60]

By 1987, the medical department was one of the most vibrant government establishments in Arunachal, nurtured from the embryonic idea and rudimentary structures left behind by the British. From 1950 onwards, the expansion of the medical department was rapid as one of the objectives of the healthcare policy was the integration of the people of Arunachal.[61] The success of this policy was reflected in the general acceptance of modern medicine by the people and the healthy growth of the population as revealed in statistical data and other socio-economic indicators. Within four decades, healthcare facilities and medical administration in Arunachal reached organizational stability and professional commitment comparable to and probably ahead in per capita terms with its counterparts in other parts of the country.

Notes

1. Civil Surgeon, NEFA to the Adviser to the Governor of Assam dated 17 May 1949, File No. Med/12 of 1949, SAGAP, Itanagar.
2. James to Rustomji dated Camp Sadiya 17 June 1948, Office of the Adviser to the Governor of Assam for Tribal Areas, File No. Med/11/48, SAGAP, Itanagar.
3. Agriculture Officer, NEFA to the Adviser to the Governor of Assam, No. GP-1/51/6983, Shillong, dated 21 December, 1951, File No. Med. 59/51, SAGAP, Itanagar.
4. Nari Rustomji, *Enchanted Frontiers: Sikkim, Bhutan and India's North-Eastern Borderlands*, New Delhi: Oxford University Press, 2010, p. 116.
5. Adviser to the Governor of Assam for Tribal Areas dated Shillong dated 21 November 1949, Notification No. A.1013/47, Medical Department, NEFA Branch, File No. 54/39 of 1949, SAGAP, Itanagar.
6. Dy. No. 940 dated 14/02/64, Office of the Adviser to the Governor of Assam, File No. P.C. 150/64, SAGAP, Itanagar.
7. Notification No. IV-8/51/8898 dated Pasighat 8 October 1951, Government of India, Ministry of External Affairs, NEFA Administration, File No. M. 92/51, SAGAP, Itanagar.
8. The total plan outlay for the first three plans is taken from Statistical Outline of North East Frontier Agency, *April 1963*, Shillong: Statistical Branch, NEFA, p. 25.
9. *Economic Review of Arunachal 1988*, Shillong: Directorate of Economics and Statistics, Government of Arunachal Pradesh, pp. 68–71.
10. *Statistical Abstract 1988 Arunachal Pradesh*, Shillong: Directorate of Economics and Statistics, Government of Arunachal Pradesh, p. 28.
11. *Census of India, 1961: Volume XXIV: North East Frontier Agency, Part II-A*, General Population Tables and NEFA Special Tables, p. 5.

12. Ibid., p. 7.
13. Barbara D. Miller, *Cultural Anthropology*, New York: Pearson Education, 7th edn, 2012, p. 175.
14. Verrier Elwin, *Philosophy*, 1957; repr., Itanagar: Government of Arunachal Pradesh, 2006, p. 8.
15. Anne Keenleyside, 'Changing Patterns of Health and Disease among the Aleuts', *Arctic Anthropology*, vol. 40, no. 1, 2003, pp. 63–5.
16. Atsuko Ibata, 'Community Mental Health and Folk Psychiatry in Tribal India', PhD diss., University of Delhi, 2014, p. 37.
17. Ibid., p. 228.
18. Ibid., p. 230.
19. *Techno-Economic Survey of NEFA: Economic Report*, New Delhi: National Council of Applied Economic Research, December 1965, p. 332.
20. *Census of India: Demographic and Socio-economic Profiles of the Hill Areas of North East India*, New Delhi: Office of the Registrar General, India, Ministry of Home Affairs, 1970, p. 242.
21. 'Policy and Objectives of Administration in NEFA', Government of India, NEFA Secretariat, 1971, File No. N.A., SAGAP, Itanagar.
22. Ibid.
23. Ibid.
24. Research Department, Government of Arunachal Pradesh, File No. Res. 96/75, SAGAP, Itanagar.
25. 'Policy and Objectives of Administration in NEFA', Government of India, NEFA Secretariat, 1971, File No. N.A., SAGAP, Itanagar.
26. 'Health plan for 1964–65 as approved by the Planning Commission', File No. P.C. 243/63 Pt. IV, SAGAP, Itanagar.
27. Chandrakant Lahariya, 'A Brief History of Vaccines & Vaccination in India', *Indian Journal of Medical Research*, vol. 139, no. 4, April 2014, p. 496.
28. 'Health plan for 1964–5'.
29. Ibid.
30. *Techno-Economic Survey*, p. 246.
31. Elwin, *Philosophy*, pp. 132–6.
32. *Techno-Economic Survey*, p. 224.
33. Ibid., p. 332.

34. Ibid., pp. 332–3.
35. 'Policy and Objectives of Administration in NEFA', Government of India, NEFA Secretariat, 1971, File No. N.A., SAGAP, Itanagar.
36. Foreign and Political Dept Proceedings, Government of India, Secret E, April 1915, Nos. 64–6, Appendix No. 2: 'Report on the Medical Arrangements on the Akha Promenade Party 1913–14, NAI, New Delhi.
37. Medical Department, NEFA Branch, File No. 11/39 of 1949, SAGAP, Itanagar.
38. Medical Department, NEFA, File No. M.91/51 of 1951, SAGAP, Itanagar.
39. 'Annual Administrative Report of Abor Hills District of NEFA for the year 1951–52', pp. 45, 94, SAGAP, Itanagar.
40. Holly Wardlow, 'Giving Birth to Gonolia: "Culture" and Sexually Transmitted Disease among the Huli of Papua New Guinea', *Medical Anthropology Quarterly*, New series, vol. 16, no. 2, June 2002, pp. 151–75.
41. J.P. Mills, Adviser to the Governor of Assam for Tribal Areas in 'Report on the Assam Tribal Areas for the year ending June 30th, 1946', SAGAP, Itanagar.
42. 'Annual Administrative Report of the Sela Sub-Agency for the Year 1951–52', SAGAP, Itanagar.
43. 'Annual Administrative Report of Subansiri Area, 1952–53', SAGAP, Itanagar.
44. R.V. Shubramanian, Deputy Adviser to the Governor of Assam for Tribal Areas, Adviser's Office to Dr J.M. Palit, CS, NEFA, Shillong, dated 3rd Sept 1949, File No. Med/19/49, NEFA, 1949, SAGAP, Itanagar.
45. File No. Med/19/49, NEFA, 1949, SAGAP, Itanagar.
46. Ibid.
47. Medical Department, NEFA File No. 90/39 of 1951, SAGAP, Itanagar; and Governor's Secretariat, File No. M-14/51, SAGAP, Itanagar.
48. 'Annual Administrative Report of the Sela Sub-Agency for the Year 1951–52', pp. 5–6, SAGAP, Itanagar.
49. Rustomji, *Enchanted Frontiers*; P.N. Kaul, *Frontier Callings*, Delhi:

Vikas Publishing House, 1976; Tarun Kumar Bhattacharjee, *Alluring Frontiers*, Gauhati: Omsons Publications, 1987; Idem., *Enticing Frontiers*, New Delhi: Omsons Publications, 1992; Idem., *The Frontier Trail*, Calcutta: Manick Bandhopadhyay, 1993; Chandra Bordoloi, *Call of the Blue Hills: Recollections from Arunachal Pradesh*, New Delhi: National Book Trust, 2012; Krishna Haldipur, *Around the Hills and Dales of Arunachal Pradesh*, NEHU: Shillong, 1985; and S.M. Krishnatry, *Border Tagins of Arunachal Pradesh*, New Delhi: National Book Trust, 2004.

50. 'Tour Diary of Dr S.B. Marak, AS (I), Mishmi Hills, Sadiya for the Month of September, October, November, December 1952 and January 1953', NEFA, Medical Branch, File No. M.29/53, SAGAP, Itanagar.
51. 'Inspection of Sepla Health Unit by Col. J.N. Ghosh, DHS, NEFA', NEFA, Medical Branch, File No. M.29/53, SAGAP, Itanagar.
52. 'Tour Notes of Lt. Vol. R.B. Sule, DHS, NEFA for Hapoli Hospital, dated 22nd March 1963', NEFA, Medical Branch, File No. M.29/53, SAGAP, Itanagar.
53. 'Tour Diary and Notes of Dr P.D. Gogoi, Offg. DHS, NEFA for the month of March 1961', NEFA, Medical Branch, File No. M.29/53, SAGAP, Itanagar.
54. Research Department, Cultural Branch, NEFA, File No. Res-25/67, pp. 14–15, SAGAP, Itanagar; and K.K. Chowdhury, DMO, Tirap District, Khonsa to the Director of Health Services, NEFA, Shillong, dated 6 July 1966, Research Department, Cultural Branch, NEFA, File No. Res. 39/67, SAGAP, Itanagar.
55. 'Tour Diary and Notes of Dr P.D. Gogoi, Offg. DHS, NEFA for the period from 13 to 19 July, 1961', NEFA, Medical Branch, File No. M.29/53, SAGAP, Itanagar.
56. 'Tour Diary and Notes of Dr P.D. Gogoi, Offg. DHS, NEFA for the period from 11 to 17 August, 1961', NEFA, Medical Branch, File No. M.29/53, SAGAP, Itanagar.
57. 'Tour Diary and Report of Lt. Col. R.B. Sule, DHS, February-March, 1963', File No. R. 48/58, NEFA/MEDICAL/1958, SAGAP, Itanagar.
58. 'K.K. Chowdhury, DMO, Tirap District, Khonsa to the Director of

Health Services, NEFA, Shillong, dated 6 July 1966', Research Department, Cultural Branch, NEFA, File No. Res. 39/67, SAGAP, Itanagar.

59. 'Annual Administrative Report of Tribal Areas of Tirap Frontier Tract for the year ending June 1951', SAGAP, Itanagar.
60. 'Annual Administrative Report of Subansiri Area, 1952–53', p. 17, SAGAP, Itanagar.
61. File No. Res. (C). 26/65, Research Department, NEFA, Cultural Branch, 1965, SAGAP, Itanagar.

4

Indigenous Perceptions on Ailments and Disease

Disease in a Frontier's History

The earliest reports about diseases and epidemics in Arunachal adduce an interesting nature of the relationship between diseases and the socio-political life of the people. An early recorded example goes back to the eighteenth century when several thousand Nyishis, reportedly under the captivity of the Ahom King Gaurinath Singh (1780–95), succumbed to the hostile weather when digging a canal for the king at a place called Kollongpur.[1] What impression the survivors carried back of the incident after they returned home to the hills can only be imagined. Oral narratives of many communities of the state are replete with anecdotes and tales of abandoned residencies in the plains because of death from 'alien' sickness.

On 2 August 1854, the touring French missionary Father Nicholas Michael Krick along with his colleague Augustine Etienne Bourri was murdered by a Mishmi villager on the Tibetan border.[2] During his first visit to the Mishmi Hills in 1851, the late priest is reported to have escaped unhurt due to his 'medical skills'. Bourri was reportedly unwell at the time of the attack and was killed on his sickbed. The attack was probably motivated by the disease Bourri was suffering from, seen as an impending sign of an epidemic that could spread to others. A certain Rungmun *Mauzadar* (revenue officer) killed by the Adis during the 1858 Sengajan raid (near Dibrugarh) had goitre; it may not be a mere coincidence that before being killed, the swelling goitre was first cut off the

Mauzadar's unfortunate neck.[3] Did the attackers consider goitre a physical impairment exported to the hills by people from the plains or was it perceived as a bad omen when confronted in a strange land? A traveller at the beginning of the twentieth century had observed that goitre was a common disease all over south-eastern Tibet.[4]

Beliefs and notions related to diseases influenced the course of the tribes' relations with the British. In 1865, a group of Adis refused to meet the Deputy Commissioner of Lakhimpur citing the prevalence of smallpox and cholera in the plains.[5] In 1883, one Lakhidar, the Mauzadar of Balipara reportedly died of fever while under the captivity of the Akas (Hrusso).[6] The incident was the immediate cause of the first Aka expedition (1883–4). Earlier, Neol Williamson, the Assistant Political Officer of Sadiya, during his visit to the Adi area had to change his route due to an epidemic outbreak. Whether the concern was the risk of contracting the disease or the fear of the official's arrival being associated with the disease, we do not have any concrete information. Williamson in his subsequent visit to the Adi area is said to have publicly insulted an influential villager's vitiligo, leading to the widely publicized murder of the visiting officer. This was the first and the only instance where a colonial frontier officer of importance had been killed beyond the Inner Line in the North-East Frontier Tract (NEFT).

The insult–retribution theory[7] behind the tragedy of Williamson's team is based on oral narratives of the people involved in the massacre and substantiated by recent vernacular work.[8] It is a different story that most of the witch-hunting history about the colonial interventions in Arunachal and contemporary government-sponsored celebrations of such incidents cast the event in patriotic garb.

Local perceptions related to disease elicited amusing reports from visitors. For example, in 1948, Ralph Izzard and C.R. Stonor, while in the Nyishi Hills in Kameng as part of the Buru Expedition, had to take care that the camera clicks were not mistaken by the people to cause measles.[9] This was because of the prevalent belief that the camera was capable of inflicting disease on the person being photographed.[10] Memoirs of many European visitors are full of similar accounts as well as about ingenuous reactions to things the people encountered for the first time: the whole village huddling together to have a glance of their 'second self' in the mirror; a haggling crowd being successfully brought to discipline and silenced by the gramophone; a companion accidentally getting killed because a curious onlooker could not resist the urge to inspect the firearm he was strictly asked to keep watch over and not touch; warriors frantically shooting at the 'strange bird' with their aconite-laced arrows as the low-flying Dakota makes reconnaissance of their territory; people refusing to be photographed lest their souls are 'taken captive'; etc.

Sickness-carrying Raids

The above examples attest to the fact that beliefs related to diseases influenced group opinions and collective actions which, at times, affected both inter-village and inter-tribe relations as well as with the frontier officials. The best-documented form of this was the sickness-carrying raid.

The earliest reference to the sickness-carrying raid was made by the English zoologist Charles R. Stonor: 'An epidemic in one village would be attributed to the disease being introduced by a man from another village, and the former would take retribution from the alleged carrier village'.[11] Stonor further expanded the explanation a decade later:

> After the outbreak of a contagious sickness the senior priest available takes the omens to decide whence it has come: the spirits reveal it to have been transmitted from another village which they name: the guilty vil-

lage being normally one with which there is in any instance a feud, or a score to be paid off: and a raid is accordingly organised to capture slaves and cattle in compensation. An influenza outbreak in the Kadeng country during 1946 led to such a procedure....[12]

The raid was an extremely retributive method to avenge the loss of life. These were usually undertaken after demands for customary reparations had failed. It led to a complex sequence of retribution and enmity among such groups for generations.

Raids were reported to be common in various parts of the globe in the generations before ours.[13] Raids from the hills of Arunachal into the plains were not uncommon since the Ahom days and the same continued even during the colonial rule in the Brahmaputra valley; most of these were not related to disease.

One of the earliest raids related to disease having important political repercussions was the Amtolla raid of 1872. G. Campbell's report attributed prevalent cholera and whooping cough in the interior Nyishi village to the raid on the administered plain village in Assam.[14] The Amtolla raid and its political fallout in the Nyishi-British relations have since been elaborated in more detail by a recent ethnohistorical study.[15] To paraphrase the details provided in the work, the incident unfolded in the following manner. There was a severe outbreak of cholera and whooping cough in the plain Nyishi villages of Gohpur and Kullungpore *mauzas* (revenue circle) in the late part of 1871. Not long after, the interior Nyishi village of Nyimte suffered heavy casualties as a result of a similar epidemic that the villagers suspected was brought by visitors from Amtolla. Parleys for settlement of the grievance of Nyimte having failed, the latter eventually undertook the raid: 2 killed, 3 wounded, and 40 taken captive. The episode raised alarm and general insecurity among the British subjects of the area and an atmosphere of intense hostility developed between the colonial authorities and the hill Nyishis. As a result, the British policy of reconciliation and diplomacy towards the Nyishis was abandoned and the policy of economic blockade and military expeditions started.[16]

The Amtolla raid was the first such officially documented incident similar to the description of the sickness-carrying raid given by Stonor seventy years later. The colonial state viewed such raids as a serious breach of order and attack on the administered territory. But from the other side, it was merely an extension of the unwritten customary decree to avenge the loss of one's kin. It involved the time-tested procedure of taking omen to ascertain the source of the epidemic and performing rituals for a successful raid.

As late as 1944, similar raids were reported from the Aka and Sajolang (Miji) area of Kameng. The incident seriously affected the peace of the whole area inhabited by the Sajolang (Miji), the Aka (Hrusso), the Khowa, and the Monpa, and understandably attracted immediate intervention from Charduar, the headquarters of the Balipara Frontier Tract.[17] One of the immediate effects of the incident was the establishment of an Assam Rifles outpost at Rupa (on the southern slope of the Bomdi la and, thus, a mountain range separated from Dirang Dzong); it emerged as the base for monitoring the Tawang situation.[18] Around the time, another incident was reported from the Aka (Hrusso) area.[19] According to Stonor, a sickness-carrying raid was the common cause for most of the (inter-village) raids.[20] And such raids were practised not only in Subansiri and Kameng but were widespread amongst the neighbouring tribes of the frontier.[21] Oral narratives generally substantiate Stonor's view but it is difficult to establish the accurate extent of this practice because only those incidents which affected the strategic interest of the frontier officials got reported; the influence of the administration and their network of village-level information did not cover most parts of the frontier until decades after the 1950s.

The two incidents cited above from official records cannot be explained in more detail lest they incite discarded memories of the recent past to be reignited. Even Stonor is silent on the above reports, about which he must, as a serving officer and an amateur ethnologist, have been aware of; even his approach to the subject is very discreet. Furer-Haimendorf had once cautioned that the identity of the informants in sensitive matters must not be disclosed.[22] Similar apprehensions might have guided anthropologists like Verrier Elwin, who described the objective of ethnography in NEFA as 'philanthropology';[23] none of Elwin's writings on the NEFA tribes mentions this practice. Even today, oral narratives relating to raids are generally transmitted to the next generation with utmost secrecy and are hardly divulged to an outsider. There is always the risk of revealing the identity of a former enemy to an outsider, who might, in turn, to cross-check, or even by mere publication of the name of the families or clan involved in the act, instigate malice.

Partly as a result of such social impediments, perceptions on disease and epidemics remained a sub-theme of religious beliefs and rituals and, thus, its effect on the local polity and customs did not attract professional investigation. Also, detailed ethnographic studies on the peoples of the state began only from the mid-1940s, by which time much of inter-clan and inter-village hostilities, the most endemic form of conflict in the hills, had significantly declined. The head-hunting tradition of some of the Naga tribes studied in detail by J.H. Hutton provides no parallel to the sickness-carrying raid of Arunachal. The nearest custom Hutton described took place in 1891 when a raid was undertaken to avert an epidemic of smallpox in Kigwema village. The raid was considered successful by the villagers, ignorant of the benefit of the vaccines previously administered to them.[24] Among the Nagas, a head-hunting raid formed a part of fertility beliefs, notions of masculinity, or a mere cycle of vendetta.[25] No practice parallel to the sickness-carrying raid of Arunachal could be found among other cultures of north-east India.

Sickness-carrying is still believed, not contrary to what modern epidemiology confirms, though the practice of retributive raid is no longer undertaken. The raids impeded social cohesion, affected settlement and migration patterns, and had an important bearing on the relations with the colonial authorities of the plains and how the hills themselves began to be approached by the state.

Between Gods and Men: The Art of Healing and Cure

The art of curing ailments and diseases through indigenous methods is a very old tradition in human history. Among the early societies, diseases were linked to 'possession by evil spirits' and spells and drugs were accordingly formulated. In this regard Gordon Childe writes:

> The craft-lore of the medicine-man, like that of the magician, had been committed to writing even in the Bronze Age and continued to be transmitted in the Iron Age ... In Greece ... there were healing gods ... who wrought miraculous cures in their temples. But outside the temple there grew up a school of private physicians who discarded the magical paraphernalia of the medicine, but not his drugs, and relied on manipulative and chemical remedies.[26]

Charles Hughes defines non-Western healing systems as 'those beliefs and practices relating to disease which are the products of indigenous cultural development and are not explicitly derived from the conceptual framework of modern medicine'.[27] The indigenous healing systems followed by the various communities of Arunachal are closely linked to religious beliefs and practices. Because of this, healing is synonymous with the traditional priest, the shaman. Disease aetiology amongst non-Western medical systems has been classified into two—personalistic and naturalistic.[28] The personalistic correlates with the shamanistic tradition (the most prevalent form in Arunachali cultures) while the naturalistic with therapeutic, as in the case of Monpa herbal healing described later in this chapter.

The term shaman is variously used along with 'native healer', 'medicine man', or 'medicine woman' depending on the cultural perspective of the writer. A performing Native American shaman and writer prefers the term 'native healer' since it represents the cultural perspective of the tradition the shaman is part of.[29] Mircea Eliade, the noted Romanian historian of religion, defined Shamanism as 'an ancient technique of ecstasy, often considered a kind of mysticism or magic but in very broad terms also a religion; for him the essence of shamanism was ecstasy'.[30] Writing about Shamanism among the Tungus of eastern Siberia, Shirokogoroff described a shaman as 'persons of both sexes who have mastered spirits, who at their will can introduce these spirits into themselves and use their power over the spirits in their own interests, particularly helping other people, who suffer from the spirits'.[31] These definitions were broadly summarized as: 'shamanism is a form of religion which centers on a magico-religious specialist who has a special ability to enter into a trancelike state at will and in the abnormal psychological state can make direct contact with the supernatural being'.[32]

Thus, the shaman was the link between the material and the spiritual worlds of the people. It is argued by Eliade that '... because the properties and conditions of the soul are within his domain of knowledge, the shaman is a curer and healer of disease'.[33] Shamanism in South Asia is classified by Jones into two contradictory types.[34] Relative to this classification, shamans in Arunachal fall within the classic type where the priest achieves a state of ecstasy, leaves their body, and travels to the netherworld. Jones argued that this kind of priest is almost absent amongst those who profess some variation of Hinduism or Buddhism. The other type of priest was dominant and was followed by those who profess a belief in the transmigration of souls.

These definitions of shaman and shamanism can be inferred to describe the indigenous priests of various communities of

Arunachal. Forster and Anderson defined ethnomedicine as 'comprising those beliefs and practices relating to disease which are the products of indigenous cultural development and are not explicitly derived from the conceptual framework of modern medicine'.[35] Among the people of Arunachal, the concept of illness was rooted in supernatural cosmology.[36] Diseases were supposed to arise entirely from a preternatural agency which can only be cured through the service of the priest through the performance of rituals.[37] Disease or ailments were the results of a breach of balance between men and supernatural forces. The shaman was the sole negotiator to safely 'retrieve' the diseased soul of a person from the offended spirits and gods.

Ailments of any sort formed an important part of this human-shaman-spirit complex. Rituals varied in nature depending on the type it was meant for. But each started after auguries had been taken, usually by checking the conjured parts of an egg, chicks' liver, etc. It is more common to describe this process by the term 'divination'. In the scheme of the indigenous belief systems, the supreme creator was presumed to have adopted a policy of non-interference in the daily affairs of the human beings and hence rituals involving diseases were not performed in the name of an absolute super-human entity. Ethno-etiology was rooted in the balance or imbalance of the human-spirit relationship and the ability of the shaman to restore it to an ideal position—a state of harmony.

Ethnographical studies on healing rites and rituals in Arunachal were largely interwoven within the study of religion and culture. As a result, the conceptual and methodical framework for the study of indigenous traditional healing practices of the state did not get much attention except for a few works done on ethnobotanical studies. Dunbar, Stonor, and Furer-Haimendorf have studied the ritual types, symbolism of the shamans' dress, and ritual structure, etc.

The shamans are known by various names across the communities of the state depending on linguistic variation. They, however, perform similar functions and fulfil the same objectives. Among the central tribes of the state, they are known as *nyubh* among the Nyishis; *nyibu* among the Apatanis; Tagin, Galo, and *miri* among the Adis. They are informally divided into various categories relative to their competence; the more proficient ones can go into trance and 'converse with the spirits'. A similar arrangement is noticed amongst the non-Buddhist communities of the state. The same system of religious belief and healing practised by the Aka (Hrusso) as reported in 1868 by Hesselmeyer[38] is still prevalent in contemporary Aka life as per recent researches.[39] Among the Nyishis, cases of cholera and smallpox were isolated in the jungle.[40] A more detailed study of the Nyishi religion, rituals, and shaman was done in 1957 under which the centrality of the shaman in healing continued to be emphasized.[41]

The Puroik who live in the midst of the Nyishis have similar religions, rituals, and priesthood.[42] Furer-Haimendorf, whose scholarship on the Arunachali tribes rests primarily on his study of the Nyishis and the Apatanis, and is still the best authority on them, observed that the religion and ritual practice of the Apatani falls in the same pattern as that of the Nyishis and the Adi.[43] The Tagin who live to the north of the Nyishis and Apatanis in Subansiri follow similar ritual practices.[44] The prominence of the shaman in the religious life of the people and the centrality of rituals in mitigating diseases are no different in the case of the Galos and the Adis living to the east and south-east of the Tagins. Ethnographic works by anthropologists confirm the similarity of cultural life and indigenous healing systems with their neighbours.[45] French missionary Father Krick and Dalton made the same observations which were later expanded by Furer-Haimendorf.[46]

In 1825–8, the Mishmis living to the east of the Adis were reported with similar religious beliefs: propitiation to various sylvan deities for the cure of any illness or misfortune and observance of ritual taboos, indicated by the sprig of a plant placed at the door to inform strangers that the house is under a ban for the time and that it must not be entered.[47] The degree and nature of isolation or seclusion during such taboo depended on the type of ritual performed. This feature is common among all the shamanistic tribes of the state. Similar propitiatory rituals of the Mishmi as mentioned by Wilcox and Needham[48] have been elaborated in more detail by recent research.[49]

In 1873, it was reported that the Khamptis, as followers of Burmese Buddhism, practised polytheistic cults and no trace of monotheism was noticed among them.[50] A similar situation was reported among the Singphos. Earlier in 1828, Neufville had noted a mixture of idolatry and superstition among the Singpho.[51] A 'Meghdeota' is also said to have been propitiated indicating the influence of religious ideas from the neighbouring plains. Macgregor and Gray also described the Singpho propitiatory rituals practised during those days.[52] The Tangsas and the Wancho, who live in the eastern part of the state, also practised propitiatory rituals.[53] These were connected to agriculture, festivals, diseases, and the welfare of human beings.

Tibetan Herbs and Bon Chants: The Monpa Healing Tradition

The contemporary healing system amongst the Buddhist communities of the state reflects the continuance of the pre-Buddhist propitiatory rituals as well as the prevalence of Tibetan medicine. This was observed when the works of a bonesetter-cum-chiropractor and a herbal expert were observed during a field visit.

Namge Tsering, aged about 65, lives in the monastic town of Tawang in western Arunachal bordering Tibet where he spends most of his days consulting and treating patients. An art learnt from whom he describes as a 'Tibetan Guruji', Namge frequently visits the nearby Pragya centre to enhance his knowledge of medicinal plants. Remuneration is voluntary on the part of the healed person. In the Buddhist healing system, remuneration is not expected and virtues like humility and selfless service are expected from healers.[54]

A thin rectangular manuscript of about thirty pages called 'Moh', written in Bhoti,[55] served as the manual for the healer. Knowledge about the time and date of start of an illness or an accident (in case of bone-fracture), the physique and gender of the patient, etc., are crucial information when consulting the almanac for choosing an appropriate course of treatment. Checking pulse at the wrist was another way of determining the course of treatment. No sacrificial rites were involved. A specific prayer in the form of a short utterance was invoked during the administering of the healing exercise. A representative healing procedure is shown in Table 4.1.

More serious ailments were referred to Tsering Tobgey, herbal specialist of Gomkhang village, located 10 km. from the town. Tobgey, who claims to have learnt Tibetan medicine from the Dalai Lama's medic himself at Dharamsala, runs a medicinal garden-cum-herbal clinic; his 'OPD' register names the top politicians of the state and army officials as beneficial clients.[56] An ex-serviceman, Tobgey laments the lack of government support for herbal medicine.

Herbal and healing experts like Namge and Tobgey are not attached to the Buddhist religious order, the Gompa.[57] Government health workers routinely approach the Gompas to request the latter to encourage the lay to seek and receive benefits of modern medicine and other healthcare facilities. It appears that amongst the Monpa, the religious order maintains neutrality in matters of methods of healing and cure and was not averse to modern healthcare interventions. Except than to inspire general virtues of service in personal and professional lives, their religion tolerates practices rooted in non-Buddhist traditions.

Table 4.1: Common Herbs Used by Monpa Healer

Ailment	*Description*	*Plant/Extracts Used*	*Method*
Bone (*Ruip*) fracture	Any kind of bone fracture	Poplar (*syarma*)	Bark of the plant used as plaster
Vein/vessels (*Chah*)	Chiropractic complaints	Titabati (*nyulum*)	A small plant; used as an anti-haemorrhage. The leaves are boiled over a small metal cup, the extracts so remaining are used to massage the affected area.
Flesh/Muscle	Chiropractic complaints	Boiled rice	Hot rice bundled into a towel, massage in the affected area
Common Illness	Common cold	Capsicum	A composite paste of *churpi* (yak's ghee, preserved for at least 13 years), capsicum, and rice is taken in portions of the size of a regular pill. The cure is claimed within a week of starting the medicine.

Source: Field study by the author. The words in italic are local names against the preceding term. Hindi/Assamese names are so reported and have not been verified.

The term *Sowa-Rigpa* ('science of healing') is being promoted to connote confusing labels like 'Tibetan medicine', 'Himalayan Medicine', 'Buddhist medicine', '*Amchi* System'—all of which refer to the same medical system.[58] The internationally cosmopolitan Buddhist medical science was enriched by other non-Buddhist medical traditions of Asia surrounding Tibet in every direction, viz., Turkic, Persian, and Kashmiri regions to the west and north-west; Indian and Nepali regions to the south; and Chinese and

Mongol regions to the east and north-east.[59] At least one authority on Tibetan medicine emphasized its origin in the ayurvedic system of India.[60] But it is also reported to embody a greater percentage of difference than similarities with the Ayurveda system.[61] Thus, there is a difference of opinion on the question of the Indian roots of Tibetan medicine.

The Monpa shaman (as distinct from the monastic lamas) have been classified by Furer-Haimendorf as *yu-min* (the oracle or magic man) who are subject to possession by gods and spirits, and who also prophesize while in trance. They are considered practitioners of the cult of local deities called *Bon* than the one inspired by Buddhism.[62] Local healing specialists like Namge are called *lah-chogan-lama* and, as can be gathered from the above discussion, they are different from the *yu-min*. A recent study by Toni Huber on Bon speaks about the worship of ancestral sky deities called *srid-pa'ilha* in the Dirang valley in Kameng.[63] While being silent on the institution of the *yu-min* and the *lah-chogan-lama*, Huber agrees that the specialists of the *srid-pa'ilha* worship fall into the shamanistic group.[64] The Pangchenpas of the Zemithang circle continued to follow their traditional healing systems even after their conversion to Buddhism.[65] Thus, we might tentatively summarize that the Monpas follow two types of healing systems—the Sowa-Rigpa system and the pre-Buddhist indigenous healing system rooted in Bon religious practices. The *lah-chogan-lama*, the herbal expert and the chiropractor, is a representative of the Buddhist healing system and the *yu-min*, the shaman, represents the Bon religious system.

From the typologies offered by Garret, Walsh, and Thupten (Shakya), the type represented by the *lah-chogan-lama* falls within the realm of medicine outlined in the classical Tibetan medical treatises. The *lah-chogan-lama* and the *yu-min* can be compared with the 'independent healer' and the 'cultic healer' of the Black Folk Medicine respectively.[66] The *lah-chogan-lama* is 'independent' as they do not owe direct allegiance to any institution while the *yu-min* derives their social meaning and ritual functions from the pre-Buddhist Bon religion.

With similar logic, they may further be compared with the Welsh natural folk medicine and magico-religious folk medicine respectively.[67] The *lah-chogan-lama*, whose healing practice is devoid of rituals except for the short incantations, relies more on the knowledge of human anatomy, use of herbs, and weather conditions. It resembles the Welsh natural folk medicine while the *yu-min* is similar to the magico-religious folk medicine. The primary tools and techniques of the *lah-chogan-lama* rely more on natural principles and objects, as also is the kind of ailments they attend to, while the *yu-min* takes up matters related to the realm of the supernatural. The contemporary Monpa ethnomedicine is an example of a cosmopolitan and eclectic healing practice. It shows strong elements of both the 'personalistic etiologies' as well as the 'naturalistic etiologies'.[68]

Herbal Healing Systems

There appears to be no clear distinction between chiropractic healers and the shaman among the larger majority of the communities of Arunachal. The recourse adopted is both ritual and 'secular' in nature. A 'soul-calling' ritual is performed in all cases of serious accidents, ailments, etc. A person is believed to have 'lost' their soul at the time of the accident or during a serious sickness and this must be profitably 'restored' before the healing can begin. This is a common practice even today in most parts of the state. Any major incident occurring in a person's life is construed to be the result of some disorder in the world of the spirit and gods in relation to that person or her/his family. Ritual intervention by the shaman was necessary to address this, along with, if any, chiropractic measures required. So, even in cases where healing from herbs through chiropractors and bonesetters are administered, ritual healing is also performed alongside. In such a scenario, while the chiropractor may be a 'secular' person, the ritual healing part is always performed by the shaman.

No indigenous name specific to herbal healers is mentioned in the extant literature, especially the bonesetters and chiropractors. Knowledge of the medicinal use of plants, herbs, and animal products formed a part of the indigenous knowledge system. A few works on traditional herbal medicine that are available are scientific rather than ethnographic.[69] The career of the herbal healer and their performances and works has not been studied exclusively. The eclipse of herbal healers by the ritual healers (shaman) in the earlier and contemporary writings could be because of many reasons.

Traditional herbal medicine did not evolve into an established system among the non-Buddhist communities because every fortune and misfortune was framed within the domain of the sacred. That there could be a 'secular', non-ritualistic approach to healing and cure has no ontological basis. The use of herbs, plant, and animal products for healing and curing emerged from exigencies of daily life and therefore remained a marginal occupation. As a result, unlike the shamans, the herbal experts did not command any distinct respect and their sole remuneration were reward for specific treatment they attended to. Being a 'secular' enterprise, herbal healing was open to any interested apprentice to pursue. The secretive way in which the experts dealt with the herbs, their composition, and their preparation restricted both the learning and the expansion of herbal medicine. Anecdotes of herbal healers of exceptional competence are common across the communities yet as a profession it is nowhere there.

The relationship between herbal and physical therapy and the sense of self-esteem about one's physical constitution, whose fate the spirits and gods guarded, is one key area which might offer a more convincing explanation on the unexplained marginality of this occupation among the shamanistic cultures of the state.

Changing Times: Indigenous and Neo-healing Forms

What is imponderable in assessing factors affecting healthcare due to the paucity of empirical data can be approached by abstract but compoundable social processes. One such area in the field of disease and healing in Arunachal is the influences of non-indigenous religions on ethnomedical practices.

The three established religious systems which have considerable influence in the state are Buddhism, Hinduism, and Christianity. The influences of the first two religions have already been noted. Vaishnavism is legally considered an indigenous religion[70] though anthropological views might differ on this. Among the Noctes and the Akas (Hrusso), the Vaishnavite faith is recognized as indigenous under the quoted law.[71] The Aka connection with the Hindu religion reportedly goes back to the nineteenth century. In 1868, C.H. Hesselmeyer, a Christian missionary writing about the Aka religion said that the concept of 'Hori Deo', a Hindu deity, was introduced by Tagi Raja, the elusive Aka warlord, among his people after he was freed from imprisonment in the plains. As a captive, Tagi had become a disciple to a Hindu guru, who in turn obliged Tagi by pledging a guarantee of the new convert's future good behaviour before the government and secured his release.[72] Going by this account, it may be argued that a civilizing element was part of Tagi's conversion to Vaishnavism.

Recent studies on the influence of Hinduism on the Mishmis and Apatanis speak about sects like the Jai-Guru and Gayatri cults being followed by sections of the respective community, but they do not offer any sociological analyses of the process.[73] Some factors suggested for the adoption of the new faiths included want of spiritual fulfilment and reasons as trivial and baffling as this: '... if purification is done through practices of other communities, the result would be beneficial'.[74] Apart from these factors, it is reported in these studies that the spread of Christianity has introduced a spiritual healing system resembling indigenous religious practices.

After the failure of early proselytization attempts in the first half of the nineteenth century, missionaries were barred from entering the state. This is an issue that has substantially been covered elsewhere in the book. After the rapid increase in the number of new adherents in the decades after the 1950s, the church gradually appropriated elements of indigenous cosmology and healing practices in their faith healing. As discussed earlier, the idea of supernatural involvement in healing from ailments and diseases was epistemologically rooted in the indigenous belief systems. This concept appears to have been exploited to suit the appeal of the new faith among the people. Speaking about the Johane Masowe Church of Zimbabwe, Englelke mentioned three things on which the former laid emphasis, viz., spiritual healing, the eradication of witchcraft, and possession by the Holy Spirit.[75] Conversion to Christianity in Arunachal is partially motivated by the fact that the church employs socially relevant meanings in the propagation and practice of their faith.

No focused study on the social processes of conversion in the state exists. Verrier Elwin spoke only of the effects of the missionary influence in the state on art forms.[76] Contemporary studies on conversion, mostly inspired by rival ideological grumblings, make superficial references on reasons like the lack of spirituality in indigenous religion and expensive ritual practices attached to it.[77] Indigenous theological aspects like the concept of soul, eschatology, perception of ghosts, spirits, and the challenging career of a shaman, etc., do not appear prominently as the primary focus of such studies. Studies on societal factors like family structure and social relations; gender issues; changing modes of livelihood; and psychological aspects could reveal deeper insights into the relationship between the indigenous healing systems and Christian faith-healing, and the process of conversion in general. For example, among the Hehe traditional psychiatrist of Tanzania, the epistemology of mental illness is developed within a belief system that emphasizes witchcraft and moral magic but the treatment followed is in the nature of pragmatic psychopharmacology, not ritual healing.[78] A similar study on the role of urbanization in psychiatric ailments among the Apatanis vis-à-vis the indigenous perception of the disease offers a fresh set of interpretations.[79]

Nevertheless, in the current exchange between the indigenous healing systems and Christian faith-healing, the latter appears to have taken the upper hand in offering a more economical and appealing healing system, at the cost of the former. The response to this overwhelming form of neo-faith-healing takes interesting turns at the level of indigenous healers while it inspires the new vocabulary of religious reform across the state. After taking a brief look at the contemporary relevance of indigenous healing systems, I offer two examples in the form of the career of two shamans to outline the predicament of indigenous healers as well as to highlight the ideological bases of the ongoing religious reform movements in the state.

A Tale of Two Shamans

Tama Mindo Romin is a renowned *nyibu* and a propagator of the Donyi Polo faith. Born in *c.*1940 at Liromoba in West Siang, he was 'abducted' by the Yapoms—a sign of a career of a shaman.[80] The Yapoms are sylvan deities who are believed to be capable of carrying away men, women, and children.[81] Young Tama, not inclined towards a ritual career, embraced Christianity in 1969 at the behest of Catholic missionaries. Five years on, the 'doting' Yapoms again abducted the new convert. Convinced that this was the final call to shaman-hood, Tama finally relented despite his adopted faith.

Uncommon for a shaman, Tama has been a teetotaller since childhood. In 1987, he helped organize the Abotani Priest Association as its first General Secretary, and presently leads the ecclesiastical wing of the Indigenous Faith and Cultural Society of Arunachal Pradesh (IFCSAP). In his long career, Tama healed many patients who did not get relief from medical interventions: one dysenteric fellow was restored to normalcy only after Tama consulted the omen and offered rituals to the *taki* (local name of dysentery) gods; on another occasion, a Sikh engineer received similar respite from a prolonged headache after the cause was traced to an offended Yapom, whose existence the government officer did not bother about when clearing a *sirek* (banyan) tree, years back during a road project.

Tadar Nyajung was a renowned shaman in the lower Subansiri region.[82] Like Tama, Nyajung kept dodging the Yapoms but to no avail. Nyajung lived with his Christian wife for about twenty years (*c.*1970–90) while he kept himself busy performing rituals. For no apparent reasons, Nyajung also became a Christian; however, he did not abandon shaman-hood. He continued to perform rituals in thorough indigenous fashion: chanting hymns; singing the origin of humans, gods, and the universe; raising ritual altars, etc., as shamans usually do. The only symbol of his conversion to the Christian faith was that he would conclude the rituals in the name of Jesus Christ. The conversion did not affect Nyajung's pre-Christian ritual routine or his reputation: needy ones kept looking for his expertise, a work he proudly continued till his last healthy days.

The two examples narrated before show how the shamans are treading the treacherous path of their careers. Tama laments the 'loss of indigenous ways of life': changing lifestyle; non-observance of ritual taboos; new food habits; new religious faiths, etc. As a result, the whole concept of well-being, confides Tama with a sense of resignation, is changing—further removed from ancestral rituals and practices. The organic idea of healing and cure stands at a momentous turn, among its practitioners and the communities. Health and quality of life are connected to concepts like harmony and balance; sickness is linked with disharmony and disequilibrium, a lack of balance between human beings and the immediate environment, including the 'forces'.[83] Speaking about the importance of food avoidance as an important element of tribal culture, one study suggested that, 'many abstentions may be interpreted as a type of primitive preventive medicine.... Not only the individual, but also the whole community may derive psychological benefits from the avoidance of certain foods'.[84]

The Donyi Polo indigenous faith movement, of which many shamans like Tama are members, responds to this challenge by adopting both the indigenous as well as new methods and ideas: shamanic hymns and songs redacted to the commoners' lexicon; minimizing the *yudum* (sacrificial offerings during rituals) and in its place opting for prayer-healing; raising prayer-cum-worship halls; weekly congregations; talks and demonstrations, etc. A recent study calls this movement 'reformist' in the 'contested domains of religious transformation'.[85] As the number of shamans declines with each passing generation, and with the institutionalization of indigenous religion, the practice of indigenous cure and healing is already undergoing a metamorphosis the full import of which can only be told by historians in times to come.

Relevance of Indigenous Healing

The efficacy of a particular healing system is not viewed from one universal criterion but is to be appreciated contextual to the culture and the region of that system. Determining the efficacy of specific treatments in any medical system is problematic—both conceptually and methodologically.[86] The indigenous cure and healing system of the state is compounded by influences from multiple directions, viz., Western biomedicine, ayurvedic, neo-religious healing, and homoeopathic systems. The outcome of this fusion may be described as what anthropologists call 'medical pluralism', which is the simultaneous prevalence and practice of many systems of medicine and healing.

Medical pluralism has been documented in many cultures similar to those of Arunachal. For example, within India, the practice has been reported from among the Muthuvans and Mannans of south India[87] and the Sonowal Kacharis of Assam.[88] The Garifuna people of Honduras—their ritual specialist is called *buaia* and they have a more developed system of natural healers like *sovador* (massager) and snakebite doctor—welcome modern medicine but at the same time exhibit a sense of confidence in some aspects of their own and do not entirely rely on modern medicine.[89] They adopted the best elements of the healing traditions of both the indigenous and modern medicines while discarding respective irrelevant elements of both. Among the Caboclo community of Lower Amazon, indigenous medicine, with a strong tradition of herbalists and midwives, is reported to be the salient marker of their ethnic identity.[90] In such cultures, modern medicine and other forces are unlikely to have an adverse impact on their indigenous medicine and healing practices.

Another example of medical pluralism is that of the Navajo people of the south-western United States. The Navajo traditionally oriented themselves geographically within a territory defined by four sacred mountains, aligned with the four cardinal points, but today they are reported to orient themselves medically in a field of vital interaction among the four modes of healing, viz., conventional biomedicine, traditional Navajo healing, the native American Church, and Navajo Christian faith healing.[91] The contemporary ethnomedicine of the Navajo people reflects the absorption and re-alignment of Christian beliefs and healing with indigenous medicine. It is important to note that the Navajo are considered one of the most missionaried people in the world[92] and live in a part of the world where the impact of advancements in modern healthcare is relatively felt more.

Access to healthcare facilities is a crucial variable in explaining why people choose one healthcare option over another.[93] But a situation opposite to this is particularly seen in the case of Andean medicine among the rural communities of Peru and Bolivia, where greater access to Western biomedicine did not lead to less prevalence of the Andean indigenous medical knowledge.[94] This shows that the relevance of both ethnomedicine and the adoption of modern medicine across cultures is not similar and not dependent only on their accessibility.

In 1978, the World Health Organization (WHO) urged the member states to foster collaboration between traditional and allopathic systems of healthcare to achieve the goals of the primary healthcare initiative.[95] This reflected the continued importance of indigenous medicine and healing system in the contemporary world as the goal of healthcare is redefined in a holistic dimension encompassing both the physical and psychological well-being of society. In contemporary Western societies, biomedicine is seen in terms of industrialized therapy which exacerbates rather than solve public health problems. As a result, popular dissatisfaction with biomedicine is reportedly increasing. This has in turn contributed greatly to the secular expansion of folk therapies throughout Western society.[96] In China, after the secularization of traditional medicine, many aspects of traditional and cosmopolitan medicine have been fruitfully integrated.[97] Indigenous medicine continues to provide succour to people as it is rooted in their belief system and culture; for example, traditional Chinese medicine considers the ailing body as part of indigenous cosmology and thus creates culturally relevant meanings to the concept of well-being.

The expansion of administrative centres, communication networks, modern education, monetization of the economy, increasing population contact, powerful cultural influences: these changes were new social experiences for the people of Arunachal. The degree of this process was described by Elwin as creating the puzzle of the impact of the atomic age on the Stone Age.[98] Despite these impacts, the indigenous rituals and healing systems continue to create meanings in the sphere of healing and well-being, to an individual and the community. Folk medicine fulfils needs that are not met by professional medicine.[99] Practices like the observation of ritual taboo and the old system of segregation of patients suffering from diseases like cholera, smallpox, bacillary dysentery, and leprosy in quickly done-up hutments away from the village have been compared with the modern system of quarantine.[100] Rather than labelling these practices as social stigma, such views create space for rational and sympathetic interpretation of indigenous beliefs and healing systems where the 'unscientific' traditions of folk healing and the science of modern medicine get the kind of consideration each deserves without disparaging the other.

Notes

1. Government of Bengal Papers, File No. 420 of 1851, ASA, Dispur; and William Robinson, *A Descriptive Account of Assam*, 1841; repr., New Delhi: Sanskaran Prakashan, 1975, p. 354.
2. Alexander Mackenzie, *The North East Frontier of India*, 1884; repr., New Delhi: Mittal Publication, 2004.
3. Bivar to Jenkins, Letter No. 99, Government of Bengal, File No. 686 of 1858–63, ASA, Dispur.
4. F.M. Bailey, 'Journey through a Portion of South-Eastern Tibet and the Mishmi Hills', *The Geographical Journal*, vol. 39, no. 4, April 1912, pp. 334–47.
5. Mackenzie, *North East Frontier*, p. 45.
6. Ibid., p. 368.
7. N.N. Osik, *British Relations with the Adis (1825–1947)*, New Delhi: Omsons Publications, 1992.

8. Onyok Pertin, *Adi Among Sim Milun E' Aabomdak Dooying*, Pasighat: Oming Pertin, 2014, pp. 55–6.
9. Ralph Izzard, *The Hunt for the Buru: The True Story of the Search for a Prehistoric Reptile in North India*, 1951; repr. California: Liinden Publishing Inc., 2001, pp. 153–4. Charles Stonor, an agricultural officer in the North-East Frontier Agency (NEFA) administration, was part of the Buru Expedition.
10. Izzard, *Hunt for Buru*, p. 109.
11. As cited in Izzard, *Hunt for Buru*, p. 109.
12. Charles R. Stonor, 'Notes on the Religion and Rituals of the Dafla Tribes of the Assam Himalayas', *Anthropos*, Bd. 52, H. 1/2. 1957, pp. 1–23.
13. J.H. Hutton, *The Angami Nagas: With Some Notes on Some Neighbouring Tribes*, London: Macmillan & Co., 1921, p. 157.
14. As cited in Mackenzie, *North East Frontier*, p. 31.
15. Tana Showren, *The Nyishi of Arunachal Pradesh: An Ethnohistorical Study*, New Delhi: Regency Publications, 2009, pp. 184–90.
16. Ibid., p. 184.
17. G.S. Lightfoot, P.O. Balipara FT, Charduar to the Secretary to the Governor of Assam dated Charduar the 7th June 1941, Governor's Secretariat, Tribal Branch, NEFA, File No. TR/24/44-Ad., SAGAP, Itanagar.
18. Ibid.
19. I. Ali, P.O., Balipara FT to the Adviser to the Governor of Assam dated Charduar the 12th February 1945, Office of the Adviser to the Governor of Assam on Tribal Affairs and States, File No. Tr. 14/45-Ad., SAGAP, Itanagar.
20. Izzard, *Hunt for Buru*, p. 109.
21. Stonor, 'Notes on Religion', p. 9.
22. Christoph von Furer-Haimendorf, 'The Presidential Address', *RAIN*, no. 18, February 1977, pp. 7–8.
23. Verrier Elwin, *A Philosophy for NEFA*, 1957; repr., Itanagar: Government of Arunachal Pradesh, 2006.
24. Hutton, *Angami Nagas*, pp. 178–248.
25. Ibid., pp. 189–262; J.H. Hutton, *The Sema Nagas*, London: Macmill-

lan & Co., 1921, pp. 160–1; and J.P. Mills, *The Rengma Nagas*, London: Macmillan & Co., 1937, pp. 16–161.

26. Gordon Childe, *What Happened in History*, Middlesex, USA: Penguin Books, 1957, p. 221.
27. As quoted in George M. Foster, 'Disease Etiologies in Non-Western Medical Systems', *American Anthropologists*, New Series, vol. 78, no. 4, 1976, p. 774.
28. Foster, 'Disease Etiologies', p. 773.
29. Medicine Grizzlybear Lake, *Native Healer: Initiation into an Ancient Art*, Illinois: Wheaton, 2007, p. xv.
30. Quoted in Kho Nishimura, 'Shamanism and Medical Cures', *Current Anthropology*, vol. 28, no. 4, August–October 1987, p. 59.
31. S.M. Shirokogoroff, *Psychomental Complex of the Tungus*, 1935, as cited in Nishimura, 'Shamanism and Medical', p. 59.
32. Kokan Sasaki, '*Shamanizumu no jinruigaku* (The Anthropology of Shamanism)', 1984, as cited in Nishimura, 'Shamanism and Medical', p. 59.
33 Mercea Eliade, *Shamanism: Archaic Techniques of Ecstasy*, 1964, as cited in Rex L. Jones, 'Shamanism in South Asia: A Preliminary Survey', *History of Religions*, vol. 7, no. 4, May 1968, p. 333.
34. Jones, 'Shamanism in South Asia', p. 333.
35. M. Forster and B.G. Anderson, *Medical Anthropology*, 1978, as quoted in James Anquandah, 'African Ethnomedicine: An Anthropological and Ethno-archaeological Case Study in Ghana', *Africa: Rivistatrimestrale di studi e documentazionedell'istitutoitaliano per l'Africa e l'oriente*, vol. 52, no. 2, Guino 1997, p. 289.
36. Verrier Elwin, *Myths of the North-East Frontier of India*, 1958; repr., New Delhi: Munshiram Manoharlal, 1999, p. 256.
37. 'Mr Robinson's Note on the Daflas (Nyishi) and Peculiarities of their Language', F/No. 420 of 1851, Government of Bengal Papers, ASA, Dispur.
38. C.H. Hesselmeyer, 'A Missionary's View of the Akas', in *India's North East*, ed. and comp. Elwin, p. 441.
39. Raghuvir Sinha, *The Akas*, 1961; repr. Itanagar: Government of Arunachal Pradesh, 1988, pp. 111–36; and Gibji Nimachow, 'Sacred Places, Beliefs, Festivals and Rituals of the Aka of Palizi Village', in

Dynamics of Tribal Villages in Arunachal Pradesh: Emerging Realities, ed. Tamo Mibang and M.C. Behera, New Delhi: Mittal Publications, 2004, pp. 219–25.

40. G.W. Dun, 'Notes on the Daflas', in *India's North East*, ed. and comp. Elwin, p. 187.
41. Stonor, 'Notes on Religion', pp. 1–23.
42. R.K. Deuri, *The Sulungs*, Itanagar: Government of Arunachal Pradesh, Itanagar, 1982, pp. 78–89.
43. Furer-Haimendorf, *The Apatanis*, pp. 131–52; Idem., *A Himalayan Tribe: From Cattle to Cash*, Berkley: University of California Press, 1980, pp. 168–73; and Idem., *Highlanders*, pp. 128–44.
44. S.M. Krishnatry, *Border Tagins of Arunachal Pradesh*, New Delhi: National Book Trust, 2005, pp. 213–19; and Ashan Riddi, *The Tagins of Arunachal Pradesh: A Study of Continuity and Change*, Delhi: Abhijeet Publication, 2006, pp. 29, 197–210.
45. Bikash Bannerjee, *The Bokars: An Anthropological Research on Their Ecological Settings and Social Systems*, Itanagar: Government of Arunachal Pradesh, 1999, pp. 153–70; L.R.N. Srivastav, *The Gallongs*, Itanagar: Government of Arunachal Pradesh, 1988, pp. 100–12; Tai Nyori, *History and Culture of the Adis*, New Delhi: Omsons Publications, 1993; and Duff-Sutherland-Dunbar, 'Abors and Gallongs', pp. 67–77.
46. N.M. Krick, 'Account of an Expedition among the Abors in 1853', in *India's North East*, ed. and comp. Elwin, pp. 236–48; E.T. Dalton, 'Capt Dalton's visit to Membu', in *India's North East*, ed. and comp. Elwin, p. 267; and Christoph von Furer-Haimendorf, 'Religious Beliefs and Rituals of the Minyong Abors of Assam, India', *Anthropos*, Bd. 49, H. 3/4. 1954, p. 604.
47. R. Wilcox, 'Rude Friends', in *India's North East*, ed. and comp. Elwin, p. 306.
48. J.F. Needham, 'Bebejiya Manners and Customs', in *India's North East*, ed. and comp. Elwin, p. 350.
49. Mills, 'The Mishmis', pp. 1–12; Tapan Kumar M. Baruah, *The Idu Mishmis*, 1960; repr., Itanagar: Government of Arunachal Pradesh, 1988, pp. 69–93; Tarun Kumar Bhattacharjee, *The Idus of Dree and Mathun Valley*, Itanagar: Government of Arunachal Pradesh, 1983,

pp. 117–42; Rajiv Miso, 'Priesthood Among the Idu-Mishmis', MPhil diss., RGU, 2005; Tarun Mene, 'Suicide Among the Idu Mishmi Tribe of Arunachal Pradesh, PhD diss., RGU, 2011; Sarit Kumar Chaudhari, 'Plight of the *Igus*: Notes on Shamanism Among the Idu Mishmis of Arunachal Pradesh', *European Bulletin of Himalayan Research*, vol. 32, 2008, pp. 84–108.

50. T.T. Cooper, 'Khampti Religion', in *India's North East*, ed. and comp. Elwin, p. 372.
51. J.B. Neufville, 'Singhpho Religion', in *India's North East*, ed. and comp. Elwin, p. 398.
52. C.R. Macgregor, 'Singhpho Rites and Ceremonies', in *India's North East*, ed. and comp. Elwin, p. 415; and J. Errol Gray, 'A Tour in the Singpho Country', in *India's North East*, ed. and comp. Elwin, p. 422.
53. Parul Dutta, *The Tangsas*, 1959; repr., Itanagar: Government of Arunachal Pradesh, 2010, p. 62; and L.R.N. Srivastav, *Among the Wanchos*, 1970; repr., Itanagar: Government of Arunachal Pradesh, 2010, pp. 79–97.
54. Ngawang Thupten (Shakya), 'Sowa-Rigpa: Affordable and Effective Traditional System of Tibetan/Himalayan Medicine for the People of Arunachal Pradesh', in *Tribal Development and Northeast India*, ed. Hage Lasa et al., New Delhi: Adhyayan Publishers and Distributors, 2013, p. 153.
55. A script used in the trans-Himalayan region. Nawang Tsering Shakspo, 'Tibetan (Bhoti)—An Endangered Script in Trans-Himalaya', *The Tibet Journal*, vol. 30, no. 1, Spring 2005, pp. 61–4.
56. Interview with Tsering Tobgey on 16 April 2015, Tawang, Arunachal Pradesh.
57. Interview with Guru Tulku Rinpoche, Abbot, Gaden Namgyal Lhatse, Tawang Monastery and Wangdi Lama of the Khinmey Monastery (Nyigmapa), Tawang on 15 April 2015 at Tawang.
58. Thupten (Shakya), 'Sowa-Rigpa', p. 142.
59. Frances Garret, 'Critical Methods in Tibetan Medical Histories', *The Journal of Asian Studies*, vol. 66, no. 2, 2007, p. 382.
60. E.H.C. Walsh, 'Tibetan Anatomical System', *Journal of the Royal Asiatic Society of Great Britain and Ireland*, October 1910, p. 1218.

61. Thupten (Shakya), 'Sowa-Rigpa', p. 153.
62. Furer-Haimendorf, *Highlanders*, pp. 169–70.
63. Toni Huber, 'Descent, Tutelaries and Ancestors, Transmission among Autonomous, *Bon* Ritual Specialist in Eastern Bhutan and the Mon-yul Corridor', in *From Bhakti to Bon*, ed. Hanna Havnevik and Charles Ramble, Oslo: Novus Press, 2015, pp. 271–90.
64. Ibid., pp. 284–5. Huber makes this conclusion keeping in view the critiques and questions about using the terms shaman, shamanistic, and shamanism to *bon*-identified phenomena.
65. Tamo Mibang and S.K. Chaudhuri, eds., *Ethnomedicines of the Tribes of Arunachal Pradesh*, New Delhi: Himalayan Publishers, 2003, pp. 108–11. A similar example in a similar society is to be found in Christoph von Furer-Haimendorf, 'Pre-Buddhist Elements in Sherpa Belief and Ritual', *Man*, vol. 55, April 1955, pp. 49–52.
66. Hans A. Baer, 'Towards a Systemic Typology of Black Folk Healers', *Phylon (1960-)*, vol. 43, no. 4, 1982, p. 331.
67. As quoted in Becka Roolf, 'Healing Objects in Welsh Folk Medicine', *Proceedings of the Harvard Celtic Colloquim*, vol. 16/17, 1996/1997, p. 107.
68. Foster, 'Disease Etiologies', p. 773.
69. Examples are Hirendra Nath Sharma, *Traditional Medicines of Arunachaand Assam: Practice & Prospect*, Gauhati: Ashok Km Sharma, 2007; Rama Shankar and M.S. Rawat, *Medico Ethno-Botany of Arunachal Pradesh*, Itanagar: Regional Research Institute, AYUSH Regional Centre, 2008; Nima D. Namsa et al., 'Ethnobotany of the Monpa Ethnic Group at Arunachal Pradesh, India', *Journal of Ethnobiology and Ethnomedicine*, vol. 7, no. 14, October 2011, pp. 7–31; A.K. Gangwar and P.S. Ramakrishnan, 'Ethnobiological Notes on Some Tribes of Arunachal Pradesh, Northeastern India', *Economic Botany*, vol. 44, no. 1, 1990, pp. 94–105; Pranjiv Goswami et al., 'Traditional Healthcare Practices among the Tagin Tribes of Arunachal Pradesh', *Indian Journal of Traditional Knowledge*, vol. 8, no. 1, January 2009, pp. 127–30.
70. Arunachal Freedom of Religion Act, 1978, Section 2 (c).
71. Ibid.

72. C.H. Hesselmeyer, 'A Missionary's View', in *India's North East*, ed. and comp. Elwin, p. 441.
73. Miso, 'Priesthood', pp. 69–70; and Hage Naku, 'Beliefs and Practices of Apatanis—Study in Continuity and Change, PhD diss., Rajiv Gandhi University, 2006, pp. 256, 264.
74. Miso, 'Priesthood', pp. 69–70.
75. Matthew Elgelke, 'The Problem of Belief: Evans-Pritchard and Victor Turner on "The Inner Life"', *Anthropology Today*, vol. 18, no. 6, December 2002, p. 3.
76. Elwin, *Art of North-East*, p. 12.
77. Nabam Tadar Rikam, 'Changing Religious Identity of Arunachal Pradesh: A Case Study of the Nyishi Since 1947', PhD diss., Arunachal University, 2003.
78. Robert B. Edgerton, 'A Traditional African Psychiatrist', *Southwestern Journal of Anthropology*, vol. 27, no. 3, Autumn 1971, pp. 259–78.
79. Atsuko Ibata, 'Community Mental Health and Folk Psychiatry in Tribal India', PhD diss., University of Delhi, 2014.
80. Information about Tama Mindo Romin was gathered through personal interview with the priest at his residence at A-Sector, Naharlagun, Arunachaon, 6 January 2017.
81. In 1855, E.T. Dalton reported about the feminine deity Yapom to be responsible for abduction of a kid in Mebo in Siang. J.F. Needham also described the Yapom as an 'evil genius' bent on harming females, and almost all the ailments which women suffer from, especially miscarriage, or ailments during menstrual period, were attributed to it (J.F. Needham, 'A Sylvan Spirite', in *India's North East*, ed. and comp. Elwin, pp. 266, 294. Countless oral testimonies of 'Yapom-abduction', some happening just months ago, are in circulation even today. These are reported especially from Kameng to Siang, where the same word is used to refer to the predatory deity. Kidnapped persons are usually traced, sometimes dead and often alive, at the humanly unreachable heights of the *sirek* branches far inside the jungle. Often, the person being carried away leaves behind their foot imprints at surprising distances; the 'retrieved' ones recount experiences of 'flying' across rivers and mountains while in

the 'sweet company' of the Yapoms. Tama also pledges to have toured some peaks of the eastern Himalayas in superhuman fashion before he was finally convinced to the 'call' to shaman-hood, a career during which the more efficient ones even take animal forms, temporarily.

82. Information about Tadar Nyojung was gathered through personal interview with the late shaman's son Tadar Nipo at the latter's residence at Doimukh, Papum Pare District, Arunachal on 7 January 2017.
83. Alver, 'Bearing of Folk Belief', p. 28.
84. Gabriella Eichinger Ferro-Luzzi, 'Food Avoidances of Indian Tribes', *Anthropos*, Bd. 70, H. 3./4., 1975, p. 417.
85. Sarit Kumar Chaudhari, 'The Institutionalization of Tribal Religion: Recasting the Donyi-Polo Movement in Arunachal Pradesh', *Asian Ethnology*, vol. 72, no. 2, 2013, pp. 259–77.
86. James B. Waldram, 'The Efficacy of Traditional Medicine: Current Theoretical and Methodological Issues', *Medical Anthropology Quarterly*, New Series, vol. 14, no. 4, 2000, p. 619.
87. K. Jose Boban, *Tribal Ethnomedicine: Continuity and Change*, New Delhi: APH Publishing Corp., 1998.
88. Farida Ahmed Das et al., 'Ethno-Medicinal Practices: A Case Study Among the Sonowal Kacharis of Dibrugarh, Assam', *Ethno-Medicine*, vol. 2, no. 1, 2008, p. 36.
89. Milton Cohen, 'The Ethnomedicine of the Garifuna (Black Caribs) of Rio Tinto, Honduras', *Anthropological Quaterly*, vol. 57, no. 1, January 1984, p. 22.
90. Mary-Elizabeth Reeve, 'Concept of Illness and Treatment Practice in a Cabolo Community of the Lower Amazon', *Medical Anthropology Quarterly*, New Series, vol. 14, no. 1, March 2000, p. 96.
91. Thomas J. Csordas, 'The Navajo Healing Project', *Medical Anthropology Quarterly*, New Series, vol. 14, no. 4, December 2000, p. 463.
92. Steve Pavlik, 'Navajo Christianity: Historical Origins and Modern Trends', *Wicazo Sa Review*, vol. 12, no. 2, 1997, p. 43.
93. Cohen, 'Ethnomedicine of Garifuna', p. 22.
94. Sarah-Lan Mathez-Stiefel et al., 'Can Andean Medicine Coexist

with Biomedical Healthcare? A Comparison of Two Rural Communities in Peru and Bolivia', *Journal of Ethnobiology and Ethnomedicine*, vol. 8, no. 26, 2012, pp. 1–14.

95. WHO Report, 1990, as cited in Nancy Romero-Daza, 'Traditional Medicine in Africa', *Annals of the American Academy of Political and Social Science*, vol. 583, September 2002, p. 174.
96. Keith Bakx, 'The "Eclipse" of Folk Medicine in Western Society', *Sociology of Health & Illness,* vol. 13, no. 1, 1991, pp. 20–38.
97. Hans A. Baer, 'On the Political Economy of Health', *Medical Anthropology Newsletter*, vol. 14, no. 1, November 1982, p. 16.
98. Verrier Elwin as quoted in Guha, *Savaging the Civilized*, p. 260.
99. Bente Gullveig Alver, 'The Bearing of Folk Belief on Cure and Healing', *Journal of Folklore Research*, vol. 32, no. 1, January–April 1995, p. 26.
100. K.K. Das, 'Health Services: Achievements and Challenges', in *Pattern of Change and Potential for Development in Arunachal Pradesh*, ed. B.B. Pandey, New Delhi: Himalayan Publishers, 1993, pp. 186–92.

5

Medicine and Healthcare in the Making of a Frontier

Not every agency of the colonial and postcolonial government interventions beget exclusive attention as medicine in establishing a friendly and lasting perception of modern administration among the people of Arunachal. From the tumultuous inter-village raids and the ever-fragile hill–plains political relationship, the hills to the north and east of the Brahmaputra found some sense of peace from the second decade of the twentieth century. The tribal polities might have exhausted their prowess against the ever-restricting and mighty colonial forces, but if one instrument of government influence did more than the gun, in the absence of the Cross, unlike most parts of the hills of the northeast, to bridge a lasting path to negotiate the new frontier into the map of the modern state, it has to be medicine.

The 1950 Earthquake Relief Operation

The greatest earthquake in the living memory of the people of Arunachal fatefully came on the evening of 15 August 1950—barely seven months after the new constitution clarified the constitutional position of the North-East Frontier Agency (NEFA) in the new order. The great shake with a magnitude of 8.6 caused destructive floods;[1] widespread disruption to traditional foot-tracks, roads, communications, buildings, and huts were reported, especially in the Lohit valley.[2] The Brahmaputra overflows its bank every year since the earthquake.[3] Sixty-six deaths were reported in the Soilang group of villages in the Mishmi Hills.[4] In northern Siang, seven houses along with twenty-three people were buried alive in Saru of Pailibo (Adi) village.[5] Communication in the entire NEFA and Upper Assam was completely disrupted for months and people were brought to the verge of starvation.[6] The destruction unleashed by the temblor was so widespread that touring officials continued to report about the destruction of the river ecosystem and agriculture cycle and productivity in the years following the disaster. Adverse effects on health and psychological impacts were also reported:

> After the great earthquake, most of the people of the district have lost the power of resistance due to the acute shortage of food or for other reasons. Various kinds of diseases which were previously unknown to the tribals made their appearance in almost all the interior villages. As a result, the number of death has gone up and few thickly populated villages are now in a dwindling state.[7]

In 1950, most of the interior villages of Arunachal were beyond the reach of the administration. The amount and extent of destruction must have been more than what officially got reported.

The earthquake happened at a time when the new government had just filled the space vacated by the British, which had belatedly started to make administrative reorganization of the long-isolated frontier. It was therefore important that a relief operation commensurate with the extent of devastation and the gravity of popular expectation from a new order was immediately carried out in a region long accustomed to the gifts from touring officials, extraction of 'ransom' (*posa*), and belatedly, medicine.

'The most extensive and elaborate civil air supply operation in the world … ', writes a former top administrator of NEFA, ' … involving the dropping by air, annually, of 25 thousand tons of supplies. … Earthquake brought NEFA to the notice of the country … we had to decline the services of volunteers on account of our inability to find accommodation.'[8] For the first time in the history of the frontier, civil airdropping of essential commodities was undertaken and till now it remains one of the largest relief operations carried out in the state. The administration also engaged scores of locals, mostly those serving in the lower levels of administration, in the relief operation; many of them were subsequently rewarded for their services.[9]

The earthquake relief operation was a testimony of the intent and humane approach of the administration in a region where, culturally, relief during individual and community distresses carried immense social value and yielded impromptu gratitude and abiding goodwill. In retrospect, the new administration dwarfed the hesitant medical works of the British with a relief work of far greater magnitude and import when a stroke of nature's fury knocked at the door of their new frontier policy.

'Allies, Not Rivals': A Medical Sociology for NEFA

Besides the few instances of initial reluctance to be vaccinated in some places, there is no reported incident of active resistance against the introduction of modern medicine and preventive healthcare interventions like vaccination throughout the state. The most important factor for this rapid acceptance and popularity of modern medicine was the intelligent policy pursued by the respective governments from the early twentieth century. Emergency medical relief and the guidelines planned for the medical staff after World War II reflected a friendly and culturally sensitive approach in the evolution of medical policy. The object of using the medicine for political ends during the colonial period was incorporated and expanded in the post-Independence period to that of the integration of the people of NEFA into the new nationhood.

The broad framework of the new frontier policy was laid in the widely known Nehru–Elwin policy of 'Panchsheel', a midway approach to tribal administration with great emphasis on autonomy and protectionism.[10] In tune with this idea, the new medical policy for NEFA was succinctly put by Elwin: 'Allies, not rivals in Medicine'.[11] It was considered important that doctors and hospitals were not seen by the people as a contender to the shamans and a sinister regime out to make the indigenous healing systems redundant. A 'medical sociology' for healthcare administration was outlined and remained the guiding principle of the expanding medical department:

> The doctors must cease to be antagonistic to the system of tribal diagnosis and cure.... A wise doctor in NEFA will make friends with the local priests, invite them to visit his hospital and let them offer prayers and make sacrifices for his patients, explaining that his own way of treatment is supplementary to theirs.... Whenever a hospital or dispensary is opened or when foundations of such buildings are laid ... the local priest should be invited to perform rites of blessing and protection.[12]

Elwin's medical sociology was inspired by an anthropologist's desire to nurture indigenous healing traditions in the face of the inevitable wave of modern medicine. This academically inspired paternalism was succinctly described by Elwin himself: 'The "philosophy" of NEFA must be built on a contended stomach, a clean skin, healthy lungs and a fertile womb'.[13] No wonder then, the evolution of philosophy for medical man was considered the most significant of all achievements during the First Five-Year Plan.[14]

Respect for local traditions was reflected in the actual practice of healthcare administration. Patients in hospitals were allowed the consolation of the tribal shamans and ritual altars were allowed to be erected in the hospital premises; charms to drive away the deities of disease were displayed in the compounds of hospitals and dispensaries.[15] Educative health posters with a local background were circulated, displayed, and explained to children in elementary schools and the outdoor patients in the health centres. In Siang, 138 potential village *yame rotung* (youth leaders) were trained in elementary hygiene and sanitation.[16]

The social stigma attached to leprosy and tuberculosis was gradually weeded out and the cured patients were rehabilitated. For example, in the early 1970s, twenty-seven lepers medically declared non-infective were sent off from the Along Sanatorium of Siang to their respective villages.[17] Attempts were made to either locate sanatoria at places where land for cultivation was available or integrate surrounding land for the same purpose so that inmates could cultivate and lead a lifestyle similar to their village life. To facilitate this, even standard sanatoria rules followed elsewhere were relaxed in deference to local customs. This was quite in contrast to a contemporaneous development in a similar region where indigenous healing was criminalized and humanitarian aid and colonial medicine were used to pathologize bodies and institute a regime of doctors, hospitals, and field matrons, all working to encourage assimilation.[18]

From the mid-1960s, medical policy began to attract renewed interest as the prime agency of national integration, understandably a result of Chinese aggression (1962). The question of the emotional integration of the people of NEFA into the national mainstream became a matter of urgent policy import:

> A sympathetic doctor will have to tell an ailing tribesman that the pills or the powder he is giving is not to bring down the temperature but to drive the spirit away from his body. It would be a good thing to class his pills 'spirit repellants'. This will create greater faith and confidence and the sick man will be more responsive to the modern treatment which will bring him closer to the culture of his developed neighbours. Doctors have better opportunities to be in closer contact with the tribal people and with a little sympathy, understanding and regard for the tribal values they will be better instruments in bringing about an effective integration of the tribal people.[19]

The passion with which this policy was pursued was reflected in two key areas: language and public media. A spirited rendering of the first has already been made in Chapter 1. In 1976, the government of the newly created Union Territory of Arunachal Pradesh produced, probably the first and only instance in the tribal North-East, a feature film, in Hindi, one of the themes of which was vaccination.[20] Attractively titled, *Meri Maa Mera Dharam*, the film was set in the early 1970s at Yazali in Subansiri. While the movie's broad intent was against conversion, as the provocative title indicates, the educative propaganda on the vaccine as the opening plot makes a clear impression of how even ideological and cultural discourse began to take shelter in the guise of healthcare. Directed by Bhupen Hazarika, and ironic for an Assamese during the times when the old wound of the Hindi–Assamese divide over NEFA had not yet healed, the motion picture has since acquired cult status amongst the people of the state and as a reminder that the route to mainstream imagination lay in speaking Hindi.

Medical Service and Racial Bias

The growing importance of medicine in establishing friendly ties with the tribes fomented ugly and the expected debate of patronage. As events folded out, the evolution of the colonial medical policy in the North-East Frontier Tract (NEFT) coincided with the period of the reforms debate (1919–35) in Assam (as in India). In an atmosphere of the reforms tug-of-war, the racial composition of the medical personnel in the hills drew the attention of both the colonial bureaucracy and the politically active elites of Assam. The question as to whether European doctors or Indian doctors, who were usually either Assamese or Bengali, should be employed in the hills began to ignite a heated debate rooted in racial prejudice, reciprocal malice, and the prospect of long-term hill–plains relations and its legacy.

To understand this debate, it is necessary to briefly reconsider the administrative background of medical services in Assam—both in the plains and the hills (including the NEFT till the 1950s). The medical personnel posted in Assam in both the military and civil establishments composed of the following categories and positions: the Indian Medical Service (IMS), the Indian Medical Department (IMD), Civil Assistant Surgeons (CAS), Military Assistant Surgeons (MAS), and Sub-Assistant Surgeons (SAS).[21] The officers in the IMS and MAS were military in training and Europeans by race who usually served on deputation in the vital and important positions under the Government of India, and in Assam, these were those in the hill districts.

In terms of qualifications and training, the Military Assistant Surgeons were inferior to the Sub-Assistant Surgeons (who belonged to the Assam Provincial Cadre) but were placed in far superior positions with better pay and allowances. This lay at the core of service anomaly much resented by the officers of the Assam Medical Service.[22] From a technical issue, the matter soon took a racial turn churning out interesting claims and counter-claims on the presumed competency and dedication to medical service, especially in the hills, and in the process, laying bare the European–Indian (Assamese) divide on the question of tribal administration.

In the early 1920s, the civil surgeoncies of the hill districts held by the European officers were proposed to be thrown open to Civil Assistant Surgeons. This was expectedly opposed by the Commissioners and Deputy Commissioners of the concerned districts, who themselves were Europeans. G.E. Soames, the Second Secretary to the Government of Assam expressed apprehension and charged the Civil Assistant Surgeons and Sub-Assistant Surgeons of inefficiency, of disliking hill posting, and not getting in touch with the hill people and securing their confidence. [23] Soames' accusation incited the Minister of Medical Department in the Provincial Government of Assam, Shri P.C. Dutta, who in return filed an extended response on the future of Assam and the hill tribes in the wake of 1919 Reforms:

Times have changed and old ideas have to be revised. … If an Indian is not respected by the Naga or other Hill tribes, it is because he has always been seen in subordinate positions. … It is the business of Indians to mix up and make friends with the Hill Tribes, take interest in their welfare. … If an Indian is so unpatriotic as to disregard these interests to avoid a little personal discomfort, he deserves no consideration. …[24]

These perceptions did not limit themselves to the particular case mentioned above but got accelerated and widened in the subsequent decades on policy decisions relating to medical administration in NEFA. The European officers' opinion on the doctors from the plains reflects a paternalistic attitude and a general distrust of plains people:

The Abor is still very prejudiced against the 'Doctor Babu' as a class. It is due to the lack of real sympathy so frequently shown by S.A.S. and which the Abor is quick to sense. That class of Government servant so often instinctively despises 'junglis' for a variety of reasons, and cannot always disguise it. There was a big deputation asking for European Medical Officer here as there used to be.[25]

In this racial and ideological tussle regarding the medical administration in the hills, the Indian doctors from the plains were also alleged to lack professional ethics. This appeared to have continued till the time the British left India as highlighted by another view on the matter:

There being very little sense of social obligation in India, the Bengali and Assamese doctor, with some exceptions, is not interested in medicine as a science, but merely as a means of financial gain. They are therefore unwilling to work in the hills where opportunities for private practice are nil, and social service is of necessity the sustaining interest.[26]

Thus, while healthcare constituted an important tool of colonial diplomacy in Arunachal and other hill areas of north-east India, the respective views of the European officers and the Assamese political class on the medical administration in the hills reflected their larger paternalistic and ideological divide. The aborted Crown Colony scheme in north-east India, retrospectively known in totality thanks to a recent publication,[27] substantiate the paternalistic views each side advocated regarding medical frontier policy in general. As a matter of subsequent debate in policy circles, it is important to note that this divide made an appearance first on the question of medical administration and hence offers a valuable prelude to the role of perception and racial prejudice in larger policymaking in the region.

Medical Minus Mission

'To the hallowed memory of those Christian missionaries,' writes H.K. Barpujari, the Herodotus of the modern history of Assam and north-east India, 'whose ceaseless toil and dedication had revived and modernised the Assamese language and literature and paved the way for Renaissance in Assam at the close of the last century'.[28] Among the 'successor' states of Assam's erstwhile hill districts—Nagaland, Meghalaya, and Mizoram—it is not uncommon to stumble upon similar tributes to the works and contribution of the missionaries in the field of literary 'renaissance', education, and medical works.[29] But no historical or ethnographic work relating to Arunachal inspiring a similar record of gratitude to the missionaries exist. The distinct history of the frontier as compared to the other hill states of the region cannot be louder.

It was not as if the land and peoples between Tibet and Assam, so crucial in Britain's geopolitical calculations, completely went unnoticed by the ever-enthusiastic missionaries. The early contacts by a couple of missionaries with some of the tribes are indicative more of individual exploratory surveys (to trace the route to Tibet) than a part of an organized attempt at medical work. Thus, we have more ethnological and very less evangelical and medical works done by the early French and American Baptists in particular and missionaries in general in the frontier. The suggestion by Krick about the pattern of the male tattoo worn by the Padam clan of the Adis as 'evidently of Christian origin' has been rejected by one prominent authority on the NEFA tribes.[30] Even as late as July 1947, the Bishop of Shillong offered the services of their Sisters in running the hospital being improvised at Pasighat in Siang and proposed on behalf of the Catholic Mission to open and run schools for the hill tribes of the then Sadiya and Balipara Frontier Tracts and to work 'earnestly for their intellectual, moral and social uplift'.[31] The request was ignored by the authorities.

Citing successive records of the American Baptist Missionary Conferences from 1890 to 1950, one study reports that the attempt to proselytize the people of Arunachal was not very successful as in the case of other hills of north-east India. The study asserts that by the 1950s some of the Adi, the Mishmi, and the Nyishi youths were converted to Christianity.[32] It is helpful to remember that such conversions were few and were achieved through educational institutions located outside the frontier; its social impacts were to be felt only in the latter decades of the second half of the twentieth century.

The unsuccessful missionary attempts in the region during the mid-nineteenth century have already been discussed at the beginning of Chapter 3. Thereafter, since the 1860s the frontier was closed for mission work.[33] The NEFT remained shut off to all British subjects (Indians and Europeans alike) after the Inner Line Regulation (1873) was enforced. Occasional passage to the area by individual travellers or commissioned explorers was strictly monitored by the government. This mechanism largely continued throughout the period of British rule in Assam until World War II necessitated a change in policy.

This explains the peculiar absence of Medical Mission in Arunachal. In Assam, the political and security reasons to 'humanize' the rebellious tribes, not so much of evangelism, had actuated the local authorities to welcome the missionaries.[34] The contrast with other hill areas of the north-east is made evident by the fact that the same agency of 'humanization' was restricted in Arunachal and in its place, medicine was experimented. The blanket absence of 'missionary hands' in the making of NEFA also explains the apparent novelty of Elwin's 'Medical Sociology' and the jerked reaction of the Union Territory administration in the mid-1970s to conversion. It is interesting to note that references to medicine and facets of indigenous healing systems come from missionary records of the nineteenth century, a period when no colonial medical policy for the frontier existed; and when it started evolving from the second decade of the twentieth century, it did so completely devoid of any missionary influence.

Medicine in the Making of a Frontier

From the Mauryan times to the present, state systems in the subcontinent had been exploiting resources in the tribal areas with the attendant process of incorporating the hinterlands to tax regimes.[35] How this process of incorporation was carried out differed from time to time, regime to regime with emphasis on one or more of the following modes: agriculture, rituals, conscription, trade, conquest, or diplomacy. Even the Vedas, particularly the earliest one, are full of accounts of contests with forest and mountain dwellers. That we read the retrospectively pejorative remarks found in the Vedic and the European colonial accounts within a context is another issue.

The process of incorporation of the hills of north-east India in the postcolonial period took the usual route that happened elsewhere in the country, which is the inheritance of the colonial legacy. Recent interpretations on the Treaty of Yandaboo (1826) question the legality of the East India Company's occupation of Assam.[36] Implicit in such interpretations is the presumed (ill-) legitimacy of Assam and Manipur in the postcolonial map of India in the context of contested questions of nationality in the region, a theme that clogs the contemporary discourse on the politics, ethnicity, and state in the region.

The Ahom state itself related with its neighbouring kingdoms, chiefdoms, and tribes, with whom it had a fluctuating overlordship over its six centuries of rule in the Brahmaputra valley. Beyond upper and central Assam, the Ahom state expanded itself in the lower valley from the seventeenth century, barely 200 years before its decline. If the legitimacy of the postcolonial state in the North-East rests on the legacy of British India's territory, the roots of contemporary disturbance and secessionist views also lie in the way the transition to colonial occupation took place and how the subsequent 'sub-nationalities' read its recent history.[37]

Interestingly, it is the farthest among such regions, the most peripheral to the state systems, the least administered, untouched by missionaries and their alleged secessionist influences which eventually emerged not only as the most peaceful state in the region but also as emotionally the closest to the Indian mainstream. It is in this story of the making of Arunachal that medicine stands, arguably, as the finest epitome of the postcolonial government's benevolent and rewarding policy.

An influential historian and a well-known biographer of Verrier Elwin credits the latter for the absence of insurgency in Arunachal: 'Elwin designed a set of policies aimed at gently easing the tribals of Nefa into their new status as citizens of India'.[38] Elwin's policy, in the biographer's view, helped most in the process of 'centring the peripheral'. This is not a lone and isolated observation. As compared to the United States, writes another, the 'Indian national policy has ... woven together a far more developed, sophisticated, and complex vision of cultural democracy and cultural self-confidence as integral to economic and political development. The Nehru-Elwin policies are remarkable in weaving into bureaucratic planning a cosmogenetic mission…'[39] Crediting the policy for creating a 'philosophic space' which helped legitimize the cultural and personal identity of the Arunachalees, it makes a profound observation that such policies 'can lay a most positive basis for future building of civic mediating structures to create a "local-national continuum" for cultural conservation and creativity'.[40] Another critique heaps a more bountiful endorsement of the policy, sounding almost satirical: 'the NEFA "Philosophy" was truly a state-making and nation-building endeavour, one of almost mystical proportions'.[41]

However, not all studies on the making of the region into Indian nationhood are as sympathetic. When Mongoloid phenotypes are yet to find a place in the common image of the 'Indian Face',[42] the exploration of the 'the Chrysalis of NEFA' and its 'metamorphosis'[43] must include the inherent lacunae of state-making and locate the place of 'emancipatory' factors like healthcare provisions in furthering the interest of the state. Just because the reigns of frontier administration passed on to a newly independent nation, the lessons learnt from colonial (non-) rule need not offer empathic wisdom in guiding policies when dealing with an ex-terra incognita.

NEFA was, as the ideological landscape in and about Arunachal stands today, probably the nearest possible example of an ideal tabula rasa in post-Independence India—lying bare for political, cultural, and lately, economic contestations and manipulations. Thus, the examples are significant: introduction of Hindi; settlement of ex-servicemen in the thinly populated areas;[44] the settlement of the Buddhist and Hindu refugees from Bangladesh; dams, illegal migration, and massive military presence;[45] and the increasing interest of the Hindu right in not only 'protection' of the indigenous faiths but in discreetly incorporating it into Hinduism.[46]

A recent review of politics in postcolonial India argues that since '...in the case of the Muslims, Christians, and other minorities their being different rendered integration impossible, no difference was conceded at all to the followers of "Indian" religions'.[47] It is within this thin margin of 'Indian' religion when the policy of integration of NEFA is read, a larger picture emerges. NEFA was devoid of missionary influences. And Christians never became a national political force in South Asia.[48] But they constitute a very influential force in the Christianized hills of the North-East. Nothing gets complete in the study of the incorporation and dissents, and by extension, the perceived 'lack' of emotional integration of the Christianized states of the north-east unless the major point of reference is Christianity and the role of the church.

While the question of the church and increasing Christianization surely provides a new and important vista for evaluation of the cultural and the ideological processes at large—an issue outside the scope of this book—it does not offer much to the analysis of the evolution of medical policy and peoples' interaction with modern medicine in Arunachal. Unlike most of the hills of the North-East Christianized during the colonial period, and as also with the Bhils of Rajasthan where the new Christians were required by the missionaries to abandon their own old beliefs in the malign supernatural causation of illness and embrace the new English medicine wholeheartedly,[49] the process of the incorporation of modern medicine in the perception of the people of Arunachal happened before education or a new religion found a similar place of influence.

Insofar as the state agents prioritized the achievement of authority over people against territory in the eastern Himalayas, the absence of the sweep of medical service across the frontier should not impede its usefulness in creating desirable impacts for respective regimes.[50] Aided by the loose and incohesive nature of tribal polities of the state,[51] opportunistic inducements, and welfare projects, however, played an important role in generating both goodwill and recruiting of local support for government interventions in the hills. 'Without the locals' willingness to negotiate', argues a recent work on the integration of the region, 'with frontier officials - to supply them, work for them, inform them—India's state presence hung by a thread'.[52] How convenient it must have been for the colonial state to opportunistically employ the method to suit its contact-when-needed policy.

Developing analytical formulations about the medical policy must be addressed within the constraints of the peculiar relationship the colonial state had with NEFA and the vicissitudes of the post-Independence state in its early decades. The common idea that the colonial incursions into the hills of north-east India were invariably intertwined with missionary activities itself needs to be understood with a new footnote now. In the case of Arunachal, the 'guardianship mindset'[53] might have marked frontier policy before and beyond India's independence but equally important is to identify how and where the patronage was exercised. And the nature of patronage was certainly going to be influenced by the intent of the 'guardian'.

With the culture of gift and communal feast inherent amongst the people of the region, what impression a particular inducement from the respective government agencies had on the people is debatable. Take the example of the *posa*. It was blackmail as well as a rightful claim of the tribes at the same time.[54] What is not debatable is that both the Ahom as well as the colonial state never used it to establish a long-term relationship with the tribes, much less integrating them and their territory. The intent of the state at this point did not require any tie with the tribes beyond checking their irritating forays into the administered plains or to facilitate occasional exploratory missions. That way, one cannot equate the *posa* with other available means of state inducements. Medicine, on the other hand, appears as a distinct medium of state mediation with the tribes; there is an implicit sense of reciprocity in that there was mutual fulfilment of the interests of both the parties—one propagating medicine and the other willing to bargain for it.

This is where the significance of medicine makes a noisy arrival. The luminous volumes of light already thrown on the Ahom–tribal and British–tribal relations, generally mournful and censorious respectively, are conspicuous in their disinterest in pursuing the means of government influences and exertion on the tribes of the region beyond the usual binary frames of analysis like love and hate, symbiotic-extracting, India-alien, etc. It is the subtle operation of capitalism and its effect on the local economy that attracts focus in the study of what an analyst calls 'colonial modernization'.[55] In such studies, mostly limited to the nineteenth century, the perimeter of colonial modernization remained limited to macro-trade analyses to show how local economies in the periphery were rendered dependent and vulnerable to the colonial market. The nature of this process is assumed to be constant, and no attempt to expand the understanding of the working of 'capitalism' in the first half of the twentieth century is made, a time when the priorities of the colonial state vis-à-vis the NEFT had changed. For example, from the twentieth century, official correspondences refer more to medicine than on *posa*—the erstwhile median of government–tribal relations.

If history is distinguished more by the 'storyness of its truth' than the trueness of the story itself,[56] then the story this book introduces about the colonial and postcolonial medical policies in Arunachal sees itself as a junior pretender on the first count while firmly rooted in the second. Irrespective of the ideological motivations of the two different states, one imperial and another nationalistic, whose medical policy this book outlines, it is in the emergence of medicine as the primary means of frontier policy and the rewarding symbol of government benevolence that the recent history of the frontier must inform itself. And during this time the NEFA awakened, entered, and acquired the consciousness, the geography, and the legitimacy of both the colonial and postcolonial state. The result is, while the dragon fumes about the dwindling candle, NEFA stole the sun's first ray to lighten the embracing motherland, as her own 'Arun-aanchal'.

Notes

1. Frank Kingdon Ward, *Himalayan Enchantment: An Anthology*, London: Serinda Publications, 1990, pp. 236–40.
2. *Census 1951 Assam: North-East Frontier Agency District Census Handbook*, pp. iv, viii.
3. Frank Kingdon-Ward, 'Aftermath of the Great Assam Earthquake of 1950', *The Geographical Journal*, vol. 121, no. 3, September 1955, p. 291. Kingdon-Ward initially says that there was little loss of life in the hills or the plains as a result of the earthquake, a statement he corrected in his book, *Himalayan Enchantment*.
4. 'Tour Diary of the Political Officer, Mishmi Hills, Sadiya, 1951', Government of India, NEFA Administration, General Department, Political Branch, File No. P-58/51, SAGAP, Itanagar.
5. 'Tour Diary of Shri B.C. Bhuyan, Political Officer, Abor Hills, Pasighat for the months of November and December, 1951', SAGAP, Itanagar.
6. Nari Rustomji, *Enchanted Frontiers: Sikkim, Bhutan and India's North-Eastern Borderlands*, New Delhi: Oxford University Press, 2010.
7. 'Annual Administrative Report of Abor Hills District of NEFA for the year 1951–52', SAGAP, Itanagar.
8. Rustomji, *Enchanted Frontiers*, pp. 116–17.
9. Government of India, Ministry of External Affairs, NEFA Administration, File No. 30/51, 1951, SAGAP, Itanagar.
10. Verrier Elwin, *A Philosophy for NEFA*, 1957; repr., Itanagar: Government of Arunachal Pradesh, 2006.

11. Elwin, *Philosophy*, p. 177.
12. Ibid., pp. 178–9.
13. Ibid., p. 61.
14. 'Policy and Objectives of Administration in NEFA', Government of India, NEFA Secretariat, 1971, File No. N.A., p. 4, SAGAP, Itanagar.
15. Ibid., p. 85.
16. Ibid., p. 87.
17. Government of India, NEFA Secretariat, 1971, File No. N.A., p. 88, SAGAP, Itanagar.
18. Mary-Ellen Kelm, *Colonizing Bodies: Aboriginal Health and Healing in British Columbia, 1900–50*, Vancouver: UBC Press, 1998.
19. Research Department, NEFA, Cultural Branch, File No. Res. (C), 26/65, 1965, SAGAP, Itanagar.
20. Government of Arunachal (Producer) and Bhupen Hazarika (Director), 1976, *Meri Maa Mera Dharam*, India: HMV.
21. Assam Secretariat, Education Department, Medical-A, March 1924, Nos. 1–12, SAGAP, Itanagar. The Indian Medical Service (IMS) was thrown open for competition from 1905 onwards (Anil Kumar, *Medicine and the Raj*, p. 133).
22. P.C. Dutta's Note dated 17th July 1923, Assam Secretariat, Education Department, Medical-A, March 1924, Nos. 1–12, SAGAP, Itanagar.
23. Soames to Minister, Medical dated 3rd October, 1923, Assam Secretariat, Education Department, Medical-A, March 1924, Nos. 1–12, SAGAP, Itanagar.
24. P.C. Dutta's Note dated 11th October 1923, Assam Secretariat, Medical-A, Education Department, March 1924, Nos. 1–12, SAGAP, Itanagar.
25. 'Tour Diary of the Political Officer Sadiya for July 1933', Assam Secretariat, Excluded Area Records, Pol-B, March 1934, Nos. 650–1674, SAGAP, Itanagar.
26. G.E.D. Walker, Political Officer Sadiya to the Adviser to the Governor dated 20th Nov 1945, Medical Department, NEFA Branch, F/No. 33/29 of 1946, SAGAP, Itanagar.
27. Syiemlieh, ed., *Edge of Empire*, pp. 1–41.

28. H.K. Barpujari, *American Baptist Missionaries and North East India, 1836–1900: A Documentary Study*, Gauhati: Spectrum Publications, 1986.
29. For a sympathetic view of the missionary history in the North-East during the nineteenth and twentieth century, see Frederick S. Downs, *History of Christianity in India*, vol. V, part 5, Bangalore: The Church History Association of India, 2003. A recent example of social history of the missionaries in the hills is that of Andrew J. May, *Welsh Missionaries and British Imperialism: The Empire of Clouds in Northeast India*, Manchester: Manchester University Press, 2016.
30. Elwin, ed. and comp., *India's North-East*, pp. 242–4. Elwin also discusses at length about the earlier attempt by Colonel R. Wilcox in 1826, after the latter discovered the use of the cross among the Padam, to trace its use to twelfth-century mission in the south of Tibet.
31. Rev. Dr S. Ferrando to the Governor of Assam dated 29th July 1947, Medical-B, NEFA Branch, File No. 80/6(c) of 1947, SAGAP, Itanagar.
32. Milton Sangma, 'Attempts to Christianize the People of Arunachal by the American Baptist missionaries (1836–1950)', *PNEIHA*, Seventh Session, Pasighat, 1980, p. 271.
33. Jenkins to Thompson, Bengal Government Papers, File No. 369 of 1861, Assam State Archives, Dispur, ASA. This restriction remained throughout the entire colonial period.
34. Barpujari, *American Baptists Missionaries*, p. 13.
35. For a recent take on this issue see Michael Gottlob, *History and Politics in Post-colonial India*, New Delhi: Oxford University Press, 2011, pp. 216–31.
36. For example, Priyam Goswami, *The History of Assam: From Yandabo to Partition, 1826–1947*, New Delhi: Orient BlackSwan, 2012.
37. Readings in this genre include that of Sanjib Barua, *India against Itself: Assam and the Politics of Nationality*, New Delhi: Oxford University Press, 1999; Idem. 'Nationalizing Space: Cosmetic Federalism and the Politics of Development in Northeast India', *Development and Change*, vol. 34, no. 5, pp. 915–39.

38. Ramachandra Guha, 'Centering the Peripheral', *Hindustan Times*, 29 April 2008.
39. Taylor, 'Public Folklore', p. 19.
40. Ibid.
41. Berenice Guyot-Rechard, *Shadow States: India, China and the Himalayas, 1910–1962*, Cambridge: Cambridge University Press, 2017.
42. Jelle J.P. Wouters and Tanka B. Subba, 'The "Indian Face", India's Northeast, and "The Idea of India"', *Asian Anthropology*, vol. 12, no. 2, 2013, pp. 126–40.
43. Chaube, *Hill Politics*, pp. 182–98.
44. Ibid.
45. Ramachandra Guha, *India after Gandhi: the History of the World's Largest Democracy*, New Delhi: Picador India, 2008, pp. 626–7.
46. The Centre for Policy Research recently published an alarming report on 'Arunachal joins the Christian northeast' (Centre for Policy Research, 8 February 2016). For a recent analysis of the religious scenario in the state and the subtle attempts at Hinduizing attempts see Sarit Kumar Chaudhari, 'The Institutionalization of Tribal Religion: Recasting the Donyi-Polo Movement in Arunachal Pradesh', *Asian Ethnology*, vol. 72, no. 2, 2013, pp. 259–77.
47. Michael Gottlob, *History and Politics in Post-colonial India*, New Delhi: Oxford University Press, 2011.
48. David Ludden, *India and South Asia: A Short History*, Oxford: Oneworld Publications, 2006, p. 243.
49. David Hardiman, 'Knowledge of the Bhils and their system of Healing', *The Indian Historical Review*, vol. XXXIII, no. 1, January 2006, pp. 202–24.
50. For the priority of achievement of authority over people against territory in the eastern Himalayas see Guyot-Rechard, *Shadow States*, pp. 263–4.
51. Dabi, 'Nation's Begotten Child'.
52. Guyot-Rechard, *Shadow States*, p. 22.
53. Benjamin Zachariah, *Developing India: An Intellectual and Social History, c.1930–50* as cited in Guyot-Rechard, *Shadow States*, p. 91.
54. The two major views on the *posa* see it either as a blackmail, an argument that originated in the days of the Ahom rulers and sub-

scribed to by many historians, or that it was offered to the tribes as their rightful claim, a view proposed by Colonel L.W. Shakeaspeare in his *History of Upper Assam, Upper Burmah and North-Eastern Frontier*, London: Macmillan, 1914, p. 106, and pledging oral narratives, by many native ethno-historians.

55. Sudatta Sikdar, 'Tribalism vs. Colonialism: British Capitalistic Intervention and Transformation of Primitive Economy of Arunachal Pradesh in the Nineteenth Century', *Social Scientist*, vol. 10, no. 12, December 1982, pp. 15–31.
56. Sudipta Kaviraj, *The Unhappy Consciousness: Bankimchandra Chattopadhyay and the Formation of Nationalist Discourse in India*, Delhi: Oxford University Press, 1995, p. 107.

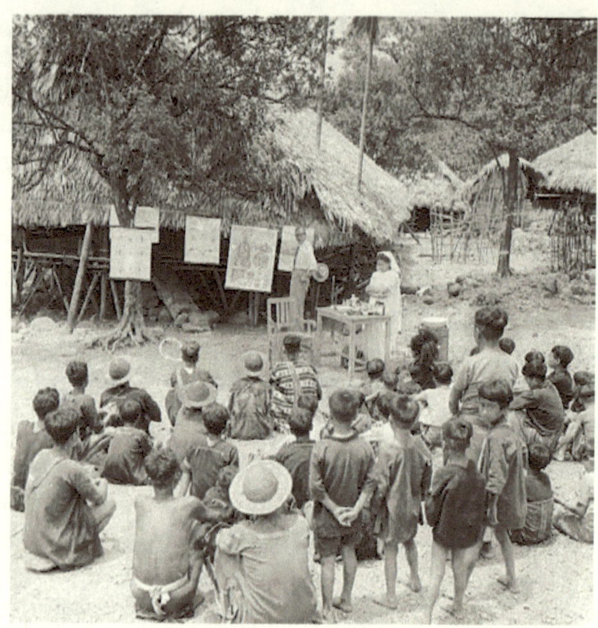

Plate 1: Health campaign in a village in Siang, undated.
Photo courtesy: Department of Information and Public Relations, Government of Andhra Pradesh.

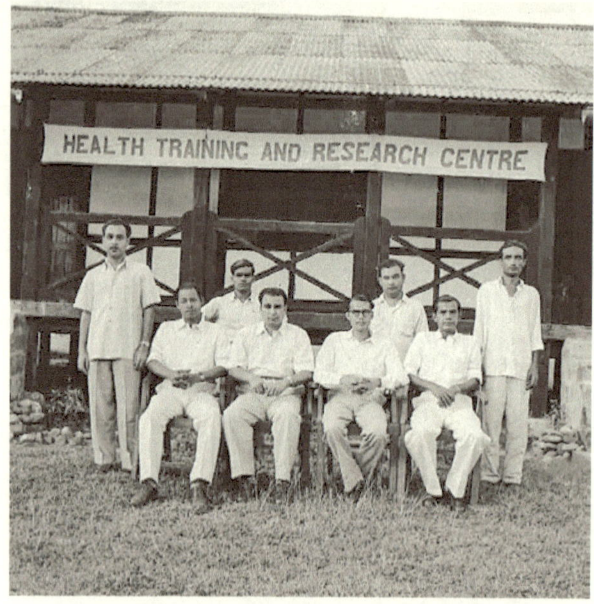

Plate 2: Medical staff training at Along, July 1957.
Photo courtesy: Department of Information and Public Relations, Government of Andhra Pradesh.

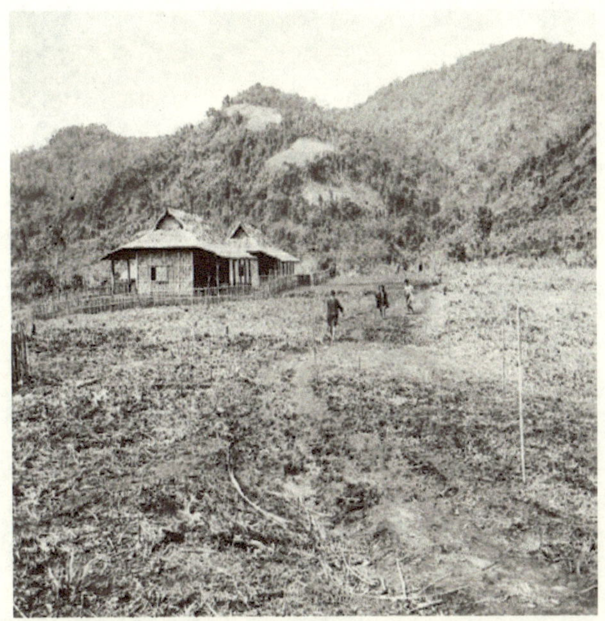

Plate 3: Newly raised hospital at Tuting, undated. *Photo courtesy:* Department of Information and Public Relations, Government of Andhra Pradesh.

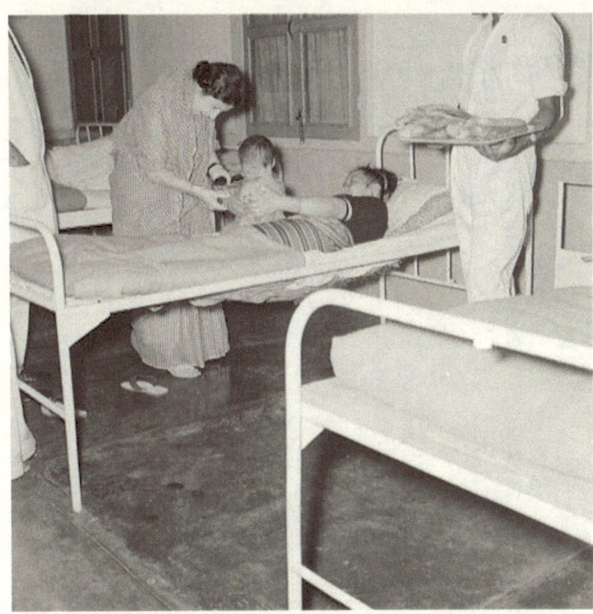

Plate 4: Mrs B.K. Nehru distributing sweets to a patient at Margherita TB Hospital, 16 September 1968. *Photo courtesy:* Department of Information and Public Relations, Government of Arunachal Pradesh.

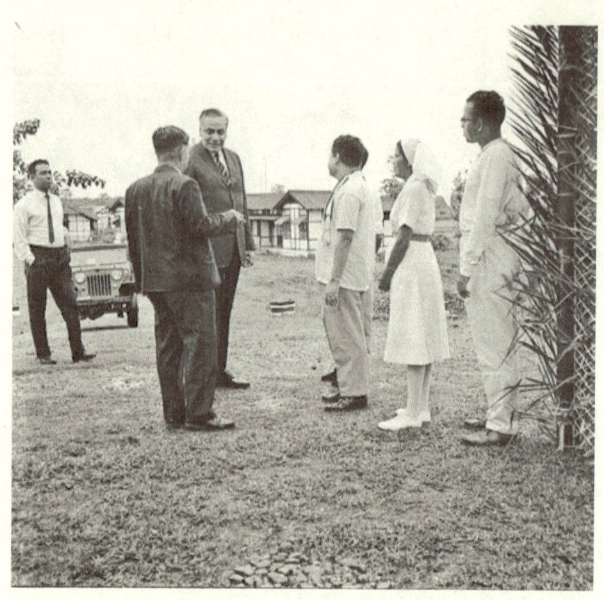

Plate 5: Governor of Assam B.K. Nehru being received by the staff of TB Hospital, Margherita, 17 September 1968. *Photo courtesy:* Department of Information and Public Relations, Government of Arunachal Pradesh.

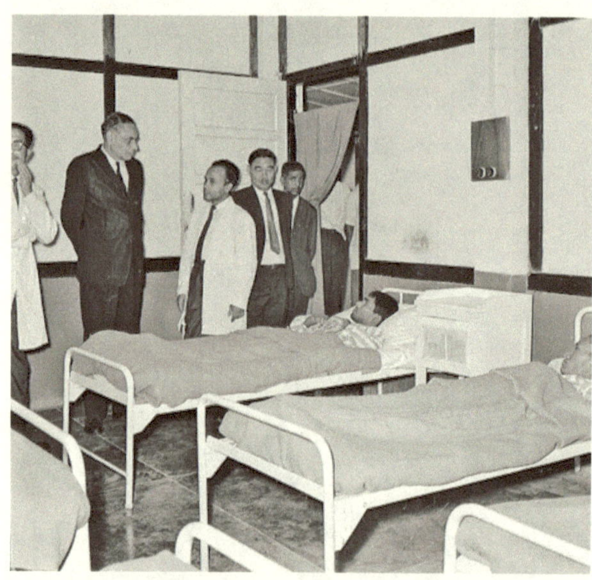

Plate 6: A doctor explaining the condition of a patient to Governor Nehru at Khonsa Hospital, 19 September 1968. *Photo courtesy:* Department of Information and Public Relations, Government of Arunachal Pradesh.

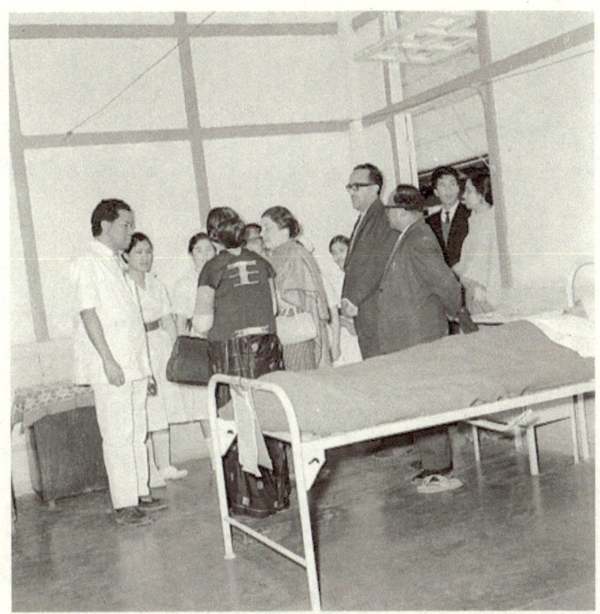

Plate 7: Mrs Nehru talking with the nurses at Pasighat Hospital, 6 December 1968. *Photo courtesy:* Department of Information and Public Relations, Government of Arunachal Pradesh.

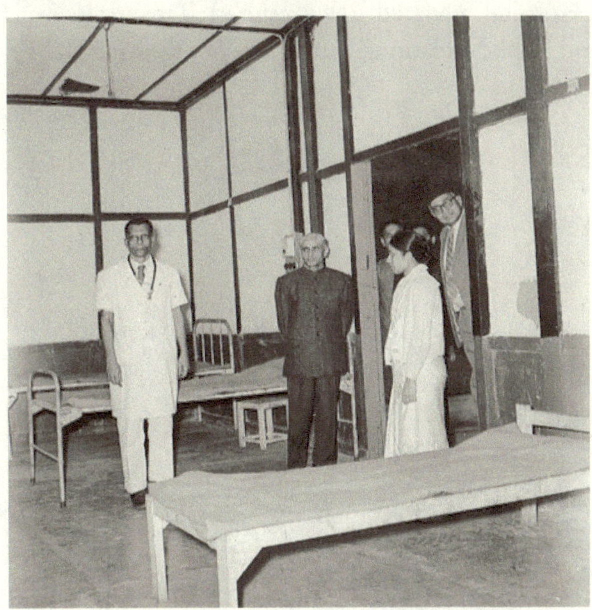

Plate 8: Cabinet Secy. & Secy. Home visiting Daporijo Hospital, undated. *Photo courtesy:* Department of Information and Public Relations, Government of Arunachal Pradesh.

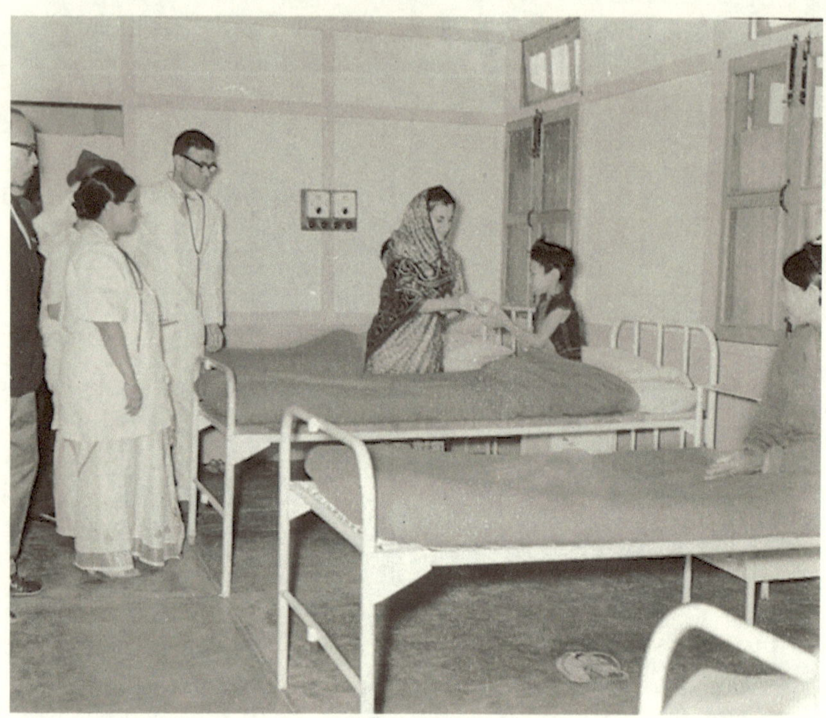

Plate 9: Prime Minister Indira Gandhi distributing fruits to a patient at Pasighat Hospital, undated. *Photo courtesy:* Department of Information and Public Relations, Government of Arunachal Pradesh.

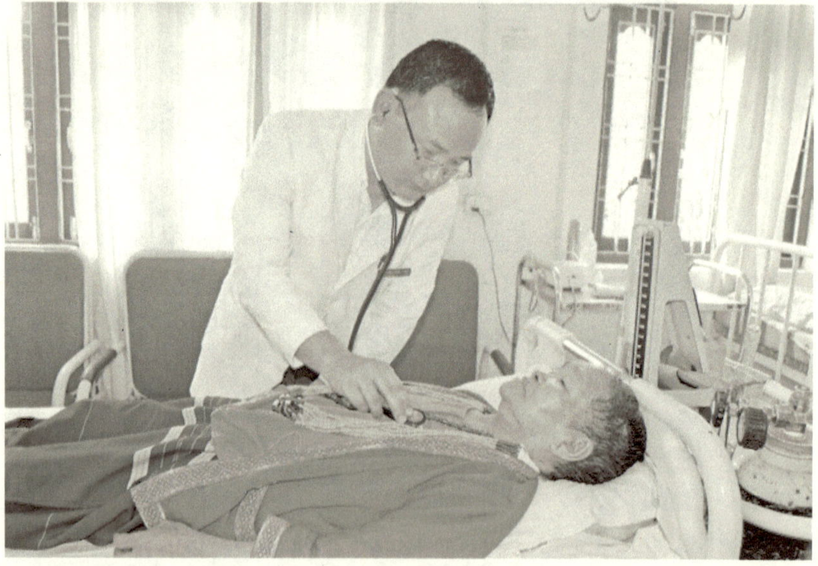

Plate 10: First-generation Arunachalee doctor treating a local patient. *Photo courtesy:* Author

Appendix I

Proposal for Expansion of Health Units in NEFA, 1945

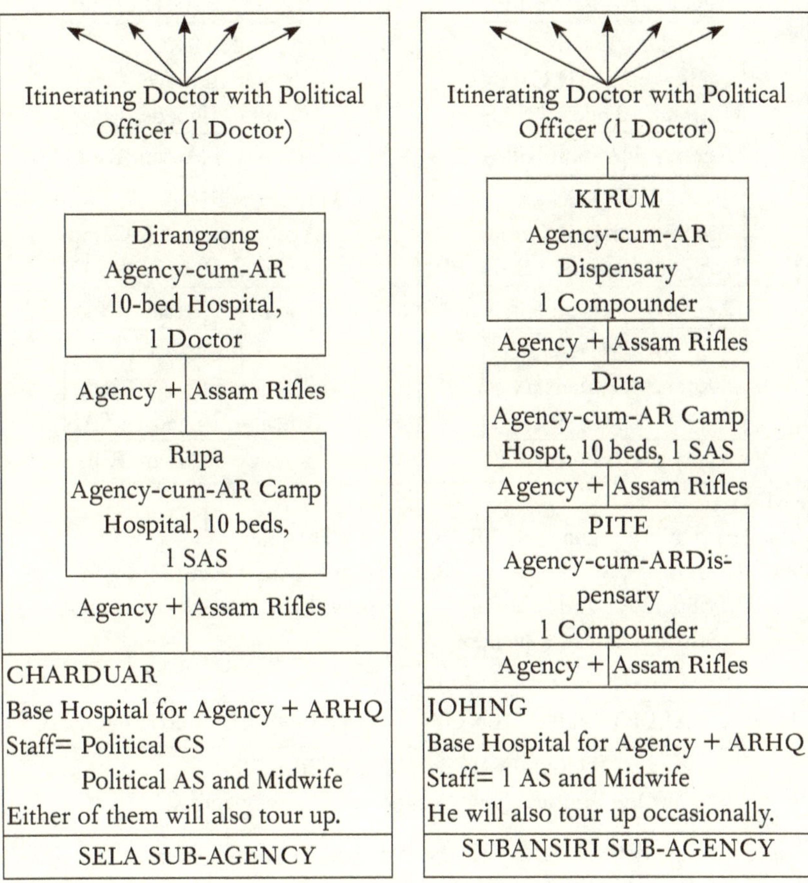

Appendix I

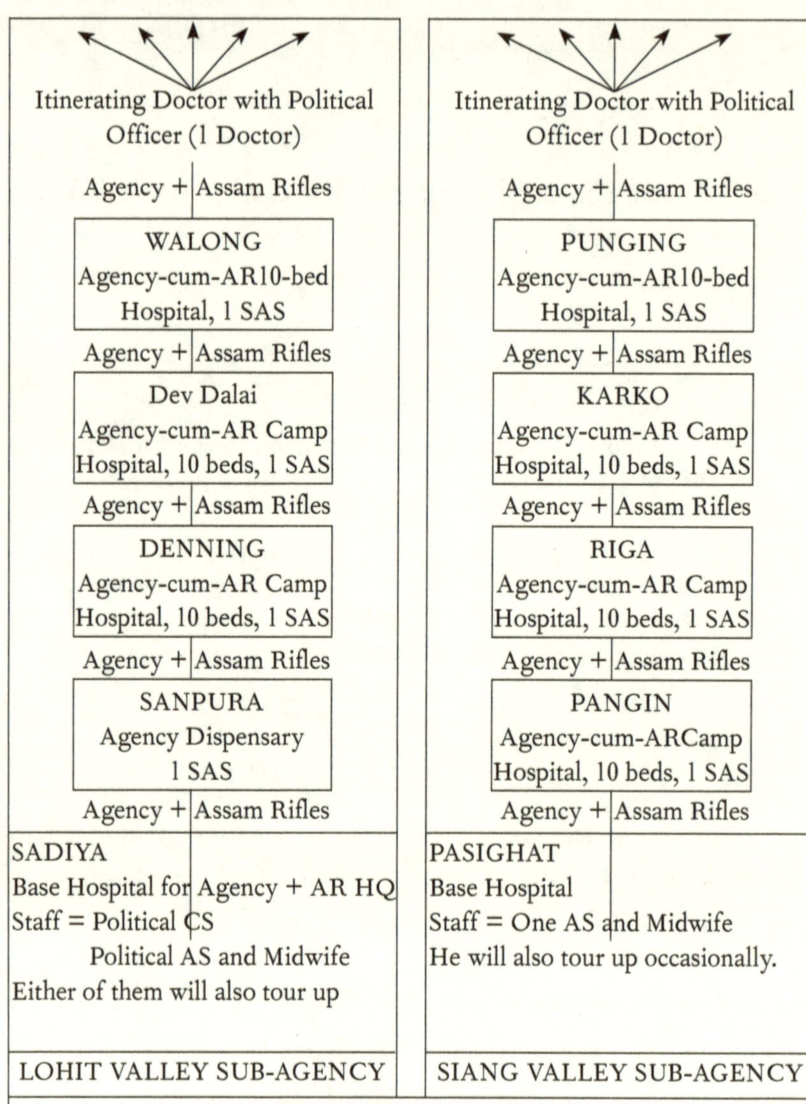

Source: Adapted from Saikia to the Adviser, Medical Department, NEFA Branch, F/No. 47/37-D of 1945, Appendix: 'Medical Scheme for NEFA, recommendations put up by the Civil Surgeon', SAGAP, Itanagar; and Assam Governor's Secretariat, Military Secretary's Office, 1945, F/No. A 1045/56, SAGAP, Itanagar.

Appendix II
Standing Orders for Doctors in NEFA, 1947

Standing Orders for Assistant Surgeons

1. Assistant Surgeons are responsible to the Civil Surgeon, NEFA for all Medical arrangements in their respective Agencies. They must remember that they are to advise the POs/APOs in all medical matters and be responsible to him so that all local orders given by him are carried out.
2. They will make frequent visits to the outposts where Medical Officers are stationed and will carry out inspections and record these inspections in the appropriate Book. Copies of these notes will be sent to the PO/APO & CS.

   Particular attention will be paid to ensure that drugs are sufficient and that he is satisfied that MOs are touring their areas. Any complaints by the MOs will be promptly dealt with and forwarded to the proper authority.
3. All correspondence relating to his Sub-agency will be forwarded by him with a note as to what action he has taken if necessary.
4. He will check all indents from MOs and satisfy himself that quantities are correct and will make necessary alterations as required before submitting them to the Civil Surgeon for countersignature.
5. At places where base Medical Stores exist he will be responsible for the care and distribution of Medical Stores and Equipment, and will take particular care that drugs required for Epidemics (Malaria and Dysentery) are readily available for use in his agency.
6. Assistant Surgeon will note that they are liable to transfer to any Sub-agency in the Tribal area.
7. They will maintain leave register of Medical Staff and inform the

Civil Surgeon when any MO has had one year's service in any one station. The policy aimed at is to transfer MOs every year (after they have had leave) to a different Station in the Sub-Agency. Every MO will in turn do a tour of duty as MO (itinerating) stationed at Headquarters.

8. Assistant Surgeon represent the Civil Surgeon and will be responsible for maintaining discipline among the Medical personnel in his Sub-Agency and in so doing will be supported by the Civil Surgeon.

Standing Order for Medical Officers-in-Charge of Hospitals in Nefa

1. Medical Officers at outposts are responsible for the Medical Care of tribal people and Assam Rifles.
2. They are responsible for the care and maintenance of drugs and equipment placed in their charge.
3. They will carry out all orders issued by the PO/APO and AS of their Agency, and will regularly tour the villages mentioned by the PO/APO.
4. They will be regularly visited by the AS of the Sub-Agency through whom all correspondence—paying bills, indents, etc., will be made. Any grievance or complaint will be reported to the AS who will either deal with it or refer the matter to the CS.
5. They will make every effort to actively co-operate with the Post Commander who is responsible for their safety. Post Commanders should be informed of their respective tours.
6. Medical Officers should bear in mind the time lag in obtaining Medical Supplies and to avoid running short and should keep a careful watch of Stocks especially drugs for malaria and dysentery.
7. MOs must realize that they are liable to transfer anywhere in the Agency.
8. All registers and stock books will be maintained by the MOs personally and will be checked by the AS and CS when on tour.

9. MOs at outposts are responsible for advising Post Commanders in all matters of Hygiene and Sanitation. Any slackness in these matters will be reported to the CS.
10. Medical Officers on tour are well advised to respect Tribal Customs, as instances may occur and have occurred where MOs have in ignorance, have infringed these customs leading to unnecessary unpleasantness.
11. Medical Officers working these newly opened Tribal areas are the PO's most useful Ambassadors, and their work is greatly enhanced if they can speak the local language. Government rewards are payable for proficiency in certain languages.

Source: Copied verbatim from Lt. Col. W.L. Neal, CS, NEFA to the IGCH dated Shillong, 8 May 1947, Governor's Secretariat, Military Secretary's Office, File No. A 1005/47, SAGAP, Itanagar.

Appendix III
Doctors Serving in NEFA, 1947

(A) Balipara Frontier Tract

Sela Sub-Agency		*Subansiri Sub-Agency*	
Dispensary/Hospital	*Class and Name of Doctor Posted*	*Dispensary/ Hospital*	*Class and Name of Doctor Posted*
Dirang Dzong A.R. Outpost Dispensary	Lt. Thantlunga, Assistant Surgeon		
Rupa A.R. Outpost Dispensary	Dr M.M. Majumdar, Sub-Assistant Surgeon		
Foot Hill (porter corps)	Dr N. Goswami, Sub-Assistant Surgeon	Duta A.R. Outpost Dispensary	Dr A.K. Bhattacharjee, Sub-Assistant Surgeon
(Base) Civil Hospital at Charduar with one doctor. Not under Tribal Area.	1 Assistant Surgeon 1 Sub-Assistant Surgeon		
Assam Rifles Hospital at Lokra	1 Sub-Assistant Surgeon		

(B) Tirap Frontier Tract

Dispensary/Hospital	Class of Medical Officer
Margrita (Base)	One touring Sub-Assistant Surgeon

(C) Sadiya Frontier Tract

Siang Valley		*Lohit Valley*	
Dispensary/ Hospital	*Class of Medical Officer*	*Dispensary/ Hospital*	*Name and Class of Medical Officer*
Karko A.R. Outpost	Dr M.N. Saikia, Sub-Assistant Surgeon	Walong A.R. Outpost	Dr Suban Ali, Sub-Assistant Surgeon
Riga A.R. Outpost	Dr C.K. Bora, Sub-Assistant Surgeon	Hayuliang A.R. Outpost	Captain Harang Buanga, Assistant Surgeon
Pangin A.R. Outpost	Dr K.M. Goswami, Sub-Assistant Surgeon	Lohit Valley Road Project/ Civil Hospital/ A.R.Outpost, Denning	Dr Paul R., Sub-Assistant Surgeon
(Base) Pasighat Civil Hospital	Lt. S.R. Marak, Assistant Surgeon	(Base) Sadiya Civil Hospital with Civil Surgeon Assam Rifle Hospital	1 Sub-Assistant Surgeon
Assam Rifle Hospital	One Sub-Assistant Surgeon One Sub-Assistant Surgeon		1 Sub-Assistant Surgeon

Source: Saikia to the Adviser, Medical Department, NEFA Branch, F/No. 47/37-D of 1945, SAGAP, Itanagar; and Assam Governor's Secretariat, Military Secretary's Office, 1945, F/No. A 1045/46, SAGAP, Itanagar, p. 14.

Appendix IV
Civil Surgeons of NEFT, 1912–1951

Sl. No.	*Name*	*Period*	*Remarks*
1.	Capt. E.C.J. McDonald	w.e.f. 29 April 1912 to 1922?	
2.	Lt. Mullins	Serving 1923	
3.	Balipara FT under Darrang CS	1923–45	Records are very sketchy; could not be traced.
4.	Capt. G.H.K. Niazi	Serving July 1945	
5.	Dr P.C. Das	Serving April 1946	
6.	Lt Col. W.L. Neal	May–June 1947	Office of the CS at Pasighat
7.	Dr A.M. Chowdhury	w.e.f. 20 June 1947	
8.	Dr J.K. Saikia	w.e.f. 11 August 1947	Referred to as 'CS' in October and 'Chief Medical Officer', NEFA in December 1951 in official correspondences.
9.	Dr B.K. Pal Chaudhari	w.e.f. 15 September 1947	
10.	Dr J.M. Palit	Serving 24 August 1949	
11.	Col. D.D. Verma	Serving on 8 October 1951	

Source: Kennedy, Officiating Chief Secretary to Chief Commissioner of Assam dated 23 May 1913, Foreign Department Proceedings, Est. July 1913 – 32–33–Part B, NAI, New Delhi; S.P. Desai's Note, Assam Secretariat, Medical Branch, Education Department, 1924, Medical-A, March 1924, Nos. 1–12, p. 16, SAGAP, Itanagar; Medical Department, NEFA Branch, File No. 33/29 of 1946, SAGAP, Itanagar; Governor's Secretariat, Military Secretary's Office, File No. A 1005/47, SAGAP, Itanagar; Medical Department, NEFA Branch, File No. 33/8 of 1947, SAGAP, Itanagar; and Government of India, Ministry of External Affairs, NEFA Administration, No. IV-8/51/8898 dated Pasighat, 8 October 1951, File No. M.92/51, SAGAP, Itanagar.

Appendix V
List of Directors of Health Service

Sl. No.	*Name*	*Period*
1.	Dr J.N. Ghosh	07.02.55 to 22.06.61
2.	Col. (Dr) R.B. Sule	23.06.61 to 24.01.66
3.	Dr W.C. Malhotra	25.01.66 to 11.12.68
4.	Dr T.P. Mukherjee	12.12.68 to 11.12.69
5.	Dr P.D. Gogoi	12.12.69 to 15.08.74
6.	Dr A.K. Bhattacharya	01.10.74 to 22.07.79
7.	Dr S.M. Mukherjee	23.07.79 to 24.08.81
8.	Dr D.K. Sengupta	11.01.82 to 24.11.83
9.	Dr J.G. Phira	25.11.83 to 29.02.88

Source: Retrieved from http://www.arunachalhealth.com/department/chronologicalchart.php , accessed 27 October 2015.

Appendix VI

Division-wise Strength of Medical Staff, 1951–1967

Sl. No.	*Year*	*Division*	*Doctor*	*Nurses*	*Mid-Wives*	*Compounder*	*Total*
0	*1*	*2*	*3*	*4*	*5*	*6*	*7*
1.	1951[1]	Kameng	8	-	-	4	12
		Subansiri	3	-	-	3	6
		Siang	8	-	2	7	17
		Lohit	7	-	-	6	13
		Tirap	5	-	-	2	7
		Total	31	-	2	22	55
2.	1952	Kameng	10	-	-	10	20
		Subansiri	6	-	-	7	13
		Siang	10	-	3	10	23
		Lohit	10	-	-	12	22
		Tirap	12	-	-	11	23
		Total	48	-	3	50	101
3.	1953	Kameng	21	-	2	12	35
		Subansiri	12	2	1	7	22
		Siang	21	-	3	14	38
		Lohit	16	-	2	11	29
		Tirap	17	-	2	8	27
		Total	87	2	10	52	151
4.	1954	Kameng	17	2	3	17	39
		Subansiri	7	1	2	7	17
		Siang	21	2	4	21	48

contd.

Appendix VI

Sl. No.	*Year*	*Division*	*Doctor*	*Nurses*	*Mid-Wives*	*Compounder*	*Total*
		Lohit	13	2	4	13	32
		Tirap	12	2	4	12	30
		Total	70	9	17	70	166
5.	1955	Kameng	10	3	3	10	26
		Subansiri	9	1	2	8	20
		Siang	18	4	5	17	44
		Lohit	11	2	4	12	29
		Tirap	15	-	2	13	30
		Total	63	10	16	60	149
6.	1956	Kameng	11	4	3	12	30
		Subansiri	9	1	2	10	22
		Siang	20	4	6	22	52
		Lohit	12	2	4	14	32
		Tirap	19	-	2	15	36
		Total	71	11	17	73	172
7.	1957	Kameng	11	4	3	12	30
		Subansiri	8	1	2	12	23
		Siang	20	4	6	22	52
		Lohit	12	2	4	14	32
		Tirap	16	-	2	16	34
		Total	67	11	17	76	171
8.	1958	Kameng	10	4	3	14	31
		Subansiri	13	1	1	11	26
		Siang	18	4	6	20	48
		Lohit	15	2	3	14	34
		Tirap	17	-	2	14	33
		Total	73	11	15	73	172
9.	1959[2]	Kameng	14	3	3	16	49
		Subansiri	11	-	3	10	33
		Siang	34	6	7	32	105

contd.

Appendix VI

Sl. No.	*Year*	*Division*	*Doctor*	*Nurses*	*Mid-Wives*	*Compounder*	*Total*
		Lohit	15	2	2	16	50
		Tirap	14	-	2	18	49
		Total	88	11	17	92	286
10.	1960[3]	Kameng	14	6	2	16	37
		Subansiri	9	3	-	12	24
		Siang	26	11	39	33	79
		Lohit	12	1	4	15	32
		Tirap	13	-	4	16	33
		Total	73	21	19	92	205
11.	1961[4]	Kameng	13	7	1	18	39
		Subansiri	9	3	-	13	25
		Siang	31	9	12	34	86
		Lohit	18	1	5	16	40
		Tirap	14	9	4	18	45
		Total	85	29	22	99	235
12.	1962	Kameng	14	4	6	16	40
		Subansiri	11	1	3	14	29
		Siang	31	1	24	33	89
		Lohit	15	1	9	16	41
		Tirap	18	-	7	21	46
		Total	89	7	49	100	245
13.	1963–4[5]	Kameng	16	5	4	16	41
		Subansiri	13	2	3	15	33
		Siang	19	3	10	16	48
		Lohit	18	4	10	17	49
		Tirap	17	4	8	19	48
		Pasighat	11	9	8	12	40
		Total	94	27	43	95	259

contd.

Appendix VI

Sl. No.	Year	Division	Doctor	Nurses	Mid-Wives	Compounder	Total
14.	1964–5	Kameng	13	3	4	16	36
		Subansiri	13	2	3	15	33
		Siang	31	9	22	27	89
		Daporizo	4	1	2	5	12
		Along	15	2	10	11	3
		Pasighat	12	6	10	11	39
		Lohit	15	4	10	16	45
		Anini	6	-	3	5	14
		Tezu	9	4	7	11	31
		Tirap	18	1	17	17	53
		Pasighat	11	9	8	12	40
		Total	88	22	56	88	254
15.	1965–6	Kameng	14	5	5	13	37
		Subansiri	13	33	4	12	32
		Siang	27	9	22	31	89
		Daporijo	3	-	1	5	9
		Along	13	3	11	13	40
		Pasighat	11	6	1	13	40+1=41
		Lohit	15	4	14	16	49
		Anini	6	-	4	5	15
		Tezu	9	4	10	11	34
		Tirap	15	2	17	17	51
		Total	84	23	62	89	259
16.	1966–7	Kameng	21	5	5	16	47
		Subansiri	13	3	4	12	32
		Siang	37	9	22	25	94
		Daporizo	7	-	1	5	13
		Along	14	3	11	11	39
		Pasighat	16	6	10	9	42

contd.

Sl. No.	*Year*	*Division*	*Doctor*	*Nurses*	*Mid-Wives*	*Compounder*	*Total*
		Lohit	21	4	14	12	51
		Anini	9	-	4	3	16
		Tezu	12	4	10	9	35
		Tirap	21	2	17	17	57
		Grand Total	113	23	62	82	281

Source: Data from 1951 to 1958 are from the *Statistical Outline of North East Frontier Agency,* April 1958, Shillong: Directorate of Economics and Statistics, Government of Arunachal Pradesh, p. 14; Data for the year 1959 is from the *Statistical Outline of North East Frontier Agency,* April 1960, Shillong: The Statistical Branch, NEFA, p. 44; Data for 1960 is from the *Statistical Outline of North East Frontier Agency,* April 1961, Shillong: The Statistical Branch, NEFA, p. 59; Data for 1961 and 1962 are from from the *Statistical Outline of North East Frontier Agency,* April 1963, Shillong: The Statistical Branch, NEFA, p. 49; and the data from 1963–4 to 1966–7 are extracted from the *Statistical Outline of North East Frontier Agency*, April 1967, Shillong: The Statistical Department, NEFA, pp. 88–89. The years are given in two consecutive year format from this period onwards, and are being shown as such.

Notes

1. Data from 1951 to 1958 are from the *Statistical Outline of North East Frontier Agency*, April 1958, Shillong: Directorate of Economics and Statistics, Government of Arunachal Pradesh, p. 14
2. Data for the year 1959 is from the *Statistical Outline of North East Frontier Agency*, April 1960, Shillong: The Statistical Branch, NEFA, p. 44.
3. Data for 1960 is from the *Statistical Outline of North East Frontier Agency*, April 1961, Shillong: The Statistical Branch, NEFA, p. 59.
4. Data for 1961 and 1962 are from the Statistical Outline of North East Frontier Agency, April 1963, Shillong: The Statistical Branch, NEFA, p. 49.
5. Data from 1963–4 to 1966–7 are extracted from the *Statistical Outline of North East Frontier Agency*, April 1967, Shillong: The Statistical Department, NEFA, pp. 88–9. The years are given in two consecutive year format from this period onwards, and are being shown as such.

Appendix VII

Chronology of Health Units, 1853–1987

Year	Place					Notes and Remarks[1]
	Siang	*Mishmi Hills/ Lohit*	*Subansiri*	*Kameng*	*Tirap*	
1853	Mebo					Father N.M. Krick's 'mobile' medical experiment
1912–15	First detailed reports on diseases					
1912	Balek/Pasighat					McDonald as temporary 2nd class Civil Surgeon
1914	Sadiya Civil Hospital					Rebuilt and expanded in 1928
1920		Charduar	Lokra			Then part of NEFT; Base of 5th AR
1921						HQ of Balipara FT shifted from Lokra to Charduar
1925?		Denning				Part of Lohit Valley Road Project; rebuilt as Civil Dispensary in 1928
1928–9			Jamiri			Opened in 1928–9; abandoned in 1930–1

contd.

Year	Place					Notes and Remarks[1]
	Siang	Mishmi Hills/ Lohit	Subansiri	Kameng	Tirap	
		Period of 'Black out'				
1940	Karko Riga	Karko health unit was shifted to Yingkiong in 1958–9				
1943				Rupa	Margerita	Itinerating doctors at Margerita
1944				Dirangdzong		
1945	Pangin					
1946	An Assistant Civil Surgeon was appointed with HQ at Charduar; shifted to Bomdila in 1955 as DMO				Tirap Gate Khonsa	
1947		Hayuliang Changwinty (Hawai) Walong Tezu	ACS with HQ at Sadiya appointed; under supervision of CS, Sadiya and Tirap FT			
1948			Foothills	Closed in 1957		
	Office of Civil Surgeon shifted from Shillong to Pasighat					
	Along Laimekuri	Dr S. Ghosh, was the first to serve in Laimekuri; entire unit shifted to Daring 1951				

contd.

Year	Place					Notes and Remarks[1]
	Siang	*Mishmi Hills/ Lohit*	*Subansiri*	*Kameng*	*Tirap*	
1949				But		
			Kimin			ACS, Subansiri Area appointed with HQ at North Lakhimpur; HQ of PO shifted from N/Lakhimpur to Kimin in 1950, and to Ziro in 1952
		Nizamghat	Doimukh			
		Dambuk	Sagalee			
		Yachuli				
						Dr K.K. Goswami first to serve in Yachuli
1950	Pasighat					Hansen Disease Sanatoriums (Leprosy Colony); the one in Pasighat was shifted to the present location from Kobo
	Along					
1951[2]	Karko				Hellgate Forest Dispensary	
	Leprosy Colony, Gungeng	Chowkham			Mobile Health Unit	
	Damro					
		Chidu				Shifted from Nizamghat due to flood of 1951
				Tawang		
	Daring	Dr S.S. Paul served from 1953–6				
	Chief Medical Officer (CMO) appointed for NEFA, HQ at Pasighat (later shifted to Shillong)					

contd.

Year	Place					Notes and Remarks[1]
	Siang	*Mishmi Hills/ Lohit*	*Subansiri*	*Kameng*	*Tirap*	
1952	Gelling	Dr S. Dutta first to serve here				
	Mechuka	Dr S. Bhadra first to serve				
	Tezu	Roing	HQ shifted from Chidu to Roing in May 1952			
		HQ of ACS, Sadiya shifted here due to shifting of HQ of Lohit district to Tezu				
				Sangti[3]	Leprosy Colony established	
				Charduar	Mobile health Units of Seppa	
				Bomdila	and Bameng converted to	
			Ziro	Seppa	regular health unit in 1955	
			(Hapoli)	Bameng	The Ayurvedic unit at	
				Buragaon	Buragaon was converted into	
					regular health unit in 1958	
1953	Mebo		Nyapin	Kalaktang		Leprosy Sanatorium
				Tawang		started at Tawang
	Gusar	Opened by Dr Kumaresh Choudhary				
1954	Basar				Namphai	Ayurvedic Dispensary in both places
	Sille					
	Daring	Mobile Health Unit at Daring opened; Dr S.K. Das				

contd.

Year	Place					Notes and Remarks[1]
	Siang	*Mishmi Hills/ Lohit*	*Subansiri*	*Kameng*	*Tirap*	
1955	Mirem					Inaugurated by Dr R. Yusuf Ali, Dy Adviser to Governor of Assam
	Tadadege					Served by D. Neog, Compounder; closed after few months
	Tuting					6 bedded unit; Dr G.N. Ganguli
			Raga (Tamen)			
1957	Manigong		Palin	Chako		Lumla Mobile health Unit converted to regular health unit in 1957
			Tali	Lumla		
1959	Liromoba		Koloriaing			
	Yapuik		Sarli			
			Huri			
1960	Gensi					
	Gasheng					
1961	Basar					

Source: The information appearing in this appendix has been generated from various sources used in this book.

contd.

Notes

1. Unless stated specifically, the information appearing in this appendix has been generated from various sources used in this book.
2. Name and place of dispensaries given in italic for this year (1951) are from Col. A.N. Chopra to Deputy Assistant Director General, Medical Store Depot, Calcutta, Letter No. 13241–44/19/41/51/EF dated the 17/8/51, Medical Department, NEFA, File No. 41/39 of 1951, SAGAP, Itanagar.
3. Office of the Adviser to the Governor of Assam Memo No. M. 92/51, Shillong 12 February 1951, Government of India, Ministry of External Affairs, NEFA Administration, File No. M.92/51, SAGAP, Itanagar.

Appendix VIII

Evolution of the Health Department, Government of India

Year	*Department*
1764	Public Department
1796	Medical service was separated into two branches— Military and Civil
1843	Home Department
1910	Education Department
1921	Education and Health Department
1923	Education, Health, and Lands Department
1945	Education Department / Health Department / Agriculture Department
1947	Ministry of Health

Source: International Council of Archives: Guide to the Sources of Asian History, India, vol. 3, no. 2, New Delhi: National Archives of India, 1992, p. 127.

Appendix IX
Towns, Population and Medical Facilities in Assam, 1901

	Towns	*Population (as per 1901 Census)*	*Hospitals in the Respective Towns and Their Capacity in Terms of Number of Beds*	*Dispensaries*
1.	Sylhet	13,891	A leper asylum	There were 135 dispensaries, out of which 35 had accommodations for in-patients. These were mainly opened at the headquarters of each district and subdivision and were being increasingly opened in rural areas.
2.	Gauhati	11,661		
3.	Dibrugarh	11,227	98 beds	
4.	Silchar	9,256		
5.	Barpeta	8,747		
6.	Shillong	8,334		
7.	Dhubri	NA	37 beds	
8.	Tezpur	NA	40 beds plus a lunatic asylum	
9.	Nowgong	NA	38 beds	

Source: B.C. Allen et al., *Gazetteer of Bengal*, pp. 42, 119–20.

Glossary

Bon	Pre-Buddhist indigenous religious form of the Monpa.
Buru	An elusive, monstrous reptile believed to dwell in swampy areas and lakes in the folklore of Tani tribes of central Arunachal Pradesh.
Duars	passes in the plains where routes and trade from the hills merged.
Lah chogan lama	Monpa bonesetter and chiropractor.
Nyiga	An adult male in Galo language.
Nyib	Shaman in Galo language.
Nyikok	In the Galo language, a person well versed in traditional rituals (but who is not a shaman), customary laws, and oral traditions. A *nyikok* is considered higher in position than the *nyib* (priest).
Nyubh	Shaman in Nyishi language.
Tani/Abotani	Mythical hero, 'first human' ancestor of the Tani tribes of central Arunachal Pradesh and upper Assam. Tani is central to genealogical history of these tribes. The Tani tribes are the Nyishi, the Apatani, the Tagin, the Galo, the Adi, and the Mishing.
Yapom	A sylvan deity bearing a feminine name commonly believed among the Tani tribes of Arunachal Pradesh to cause different kinds of illness, especially miscarriage.

Yudum	Sacrificial offerings in the form of animals in the indigenous ritual.
Yu-min	Monpa equivalent of *nyub* (shaman); representative of the *Bon* religion.

Bibliography

Archival Records

Assam State Archives, Dispur, Guwahati

Assam Secretariat Correspondences and Proceedings
Government of Bengal Papers
Municipal Department Correspondences

National Archives of India, New Delhi

Foreign and Political Department Proceedings
Foreign Department Proceedings
Home Department Proceedings

State Archives, Government of Arunachal Pradesh, Itanagar

Annual Administrative Reports
Assam Governor's Secretariat, Military Secretary's Office
Assam Secretariat Proceedings, Excluded Areas Records
Assam Secretariat, Education Department Notes
Assam Secretariat, Medical-A, Medical-B Correspondences
Government of India, NEFA Secretariat
Governor's Secretariat, Excluded Areas Records
Medical Department, NEFA Branch Records
NEFA, Medical Branch Records

Office of the Adviser to the Governor of Assam on Tribal Affairs – Reports, Records and Correspondences
Personal Files
Planning Commission Correspondences
Report on the Assam Tribal Areas
Research Department Files, NEFA
Tour Dairies and Notes

Audio-Visual Sources

Government of Arunachal Pradesh (Producer) and Bhupen Hazarika (Director), 1976, *Meri Maa Mera Dharam*, India, HMV. Retrieved from: https://www.youtube.com/watch?v=giSCilYe378, accessed 7 February 2016.

Articles from Journals, Proceedings, Books, and Newspapers

Alver, BenteGullveig, 'The Bearing of Folk Belief on Cure and Healing', *Journal of Folklore Research*, vol. 32, no. 1, January–April 1995, pp. 21–33.

Anquandah, James, 'African Ethnomedicine: An Anthropological and Ethno-archaeological Case Study in Ghana', *Africa: Rivistatrimestrale di studi e documentazionedell'istitutoitaliano per l'Africa e l'oriente,* Anno 52, no. 2, Guino 1997, pp. 289–98.

Ansari, Tahir Hussain, 'Disease and Medicine in the Colonial Assam during 19th Century', *Journal of Business Management & Social Sciences Research (JBM&SSR),* vol. 2, no. 1, January 2013, pp. 92–6.

Axtell, James, 'Ethnohistory: An Historian's Viewpoint', *Ethnohistory*, vol. 26, no. 1, Winter 1979, pp. 1–13.

Baer, Hans, A., 'On the Political Economy of Health', *Medical Anthropology Newsletter*, vol. 14, no. 1, November 1982, pp. 1–2, 13–17.

Bibliography

Baer, Hans, A., 'Towards a Systemic Typology of Black Folk Healers', *Phylon (1960-)*, vol. 43, no. 4, 4th Qtr. 1982, pp. 327–43.

Bailey, F.M., 'Journey Through a Portion of South-Eastern Tibet and the Mishmi Hills', *The Geographical Journal*, vol. 39, no. 4, April 1912, pp. 334–47.

Bakx, Keith, 'The "Eclipse" of Folk Medicine in Western Society', *Sociology of Health & Illness*, vol. 13, no. 1, 1991, pp. 20–38.

Barua, Sanjib, 'Nationalizing Space: Cosmetic Federalism and the Politics of Development in Northeast India', *Development and Change*, vol. 34, no. 5, 2003, pp. 915–39.

Bjerken, Zeff, 'Exorcising the Illusions of *Bon* "Shamans": A Critical Genealogy of Shamanism in Tibetan Religions', *Revue d'etudestibetaines*, vol. 6, 2004, pp. 4–59.

Blackburn, Stuart, 'Memories of Migration: Notes on Legends and Beads in Arunachal Pradesh, India', *European Bulletin of Himalayan Research*, vol. 25/26, 2003/2004, pp. 16–60.

Bora, Shiela, 'American Baptist Missionaries' Ethnological Writings: The Singphos and the Namsang Nagas', in *Pre-Colonial History and Traditions of Arunachal Pradesh*, ed. Sudhir Kumar Singh and Ashan Riddi, Guwahati: DVS Publishers, 2017, pp. 314–42.

Chaudhari, Sarit Kumar, 'Plight of the *Igus*: Notes on Shamanism among the Idu Mishmis of Arunachal Pradesh', *European Bulletin of Himalayan Research*, vol. 32, 2008, pp. 84–108.

Chaudhari, Sarit Kumar, 'The Institutionalization of Tribal Religion: Recasting the Donyi-Polo Movement in Arunachal Pradesh', *Asian Ethnology*, vol. 72, no. 2, 2013, pp. 259–77.

Chaudhary, J.N., 'Post-Colonial Policy towards Ethnic Minorities of North-East India (A Comparative Approach) with Special Reference to Arunachal Pradesh', in *Nationality, Ethnicity, and Cultural Identity in North-East India*, ed. B. Pakem, Guwahati and New Delhi: Omsons Publications, 1990, pp. 127–45.

Cohen, Milton, 'The Ethnomedicine of the Garifuna (Black Caribs) of Rio Tinto, Honduras', *Anthropological Quaterly*, vol. 57, no. 1, January 1984, pp. 16–27.

Csordas, Thomas J., 'The Navajo Healing Project', *Medical Anthro-*

pology Quarterly, New Series, vol. 14, no. 4, December 2000, pp. 463–75.

Dabi, Tajen, 'A Nation's Begotten Child: Arunachal Pradesh in India's Troubled Northeast', in *Development and Ethnicity in northeast India*, ed. Komol Singha and M. Amarjeet Singh, New Delhi: Routledge, 2016, pp. 213–25.

Das, Farida Ahmed, Indira Barua, and Deepanjana Dutta Das, 'Ethno-Medicinal Practices: A Case Study among the Sonowal Kacharis of Dibrugarh, Assam', *Ethno-Medicine*, vol. 2, no. 1, 2008, pp. 33–7.

Das, K.K., 'Health Services: Achievements and Challenges', in *Pattern of Change and Potential for Development in Arunachal Pradesh*, ed. B.B. Pandey, New Delhi: Himalayan Publishers, 1993, pp. 186–92.

Dawar, Jagdish Lal, 'Literary Production and Social Reality in Arunachal Pradesh: Representation of Marriage Systems of Galo Adi in Lumma Dai's *Konyar-Mulya*', *Proceedings of the North East India History Association*, 21st Session, Imphal, 2011, pp. 244–57.

Dawar, Jagdish Lal, 'Religious Conversion in Arunachal Pradesh since 1950s: A Study of Perceptions', *Proceedings of the North East India History Association*, 20th Session, Dibrugarh, 2000, pp. 300–4.

Deka, Harekrishna, 'North-east in Fragments and Invention of a Metaphor', in *Souvenir of the North East India History Association*, ed. Chandan Kumar Sharma, 29th Annual Session, Dibrugarh, 2008, pp. 101–13.

Dhar, Bibash, 'Tribal Identity Dilemma in Arunachal Pradesh', in *Nationality, Ethnicity and Cultural Identity in Norht-East India*, ed. B. Pakem, Guwahati and New Delhi: Omsons Publications, 1990, pp. 121–6.

Duff-Sutherland-Dunbar, George, 'Abors and Gallongs: Notes on Certain Hill Tribes of the Indo-Tibetan Border', *Memoirs of Asiatic Society of Bengal*, vol. 5, extra no., 1915, pp. 1–91.

Dutta, Binayak, 'Constructing India's North Eastern Tribal Policy and Verrier Elwin—A Review', *Proceedings of the North East India History Association*, 19th Session, Kohima, 1999, pp. 288–96.

Edgerton, Robert B., 'A Traditional African Psychiatrist', *Southwestern Journal of Anthropology*, vol. 27, no. 3, Autumn 1971, pp. 259–78.

Elgelke, Matthew, 'The Problem of Belief: Evans-Pritchard and Victor Turner on "The Inner Life"', *Anthropology Today*, vol. 18, no. 6, December 2002, pp. 3–8.

Fabrega, Jr., Horacio, 'Earliest Phases in the Evolution of Sickness and Healing', *Medical Anthropology Quarterly*, New Series, vol. 11, no. 1, March 1997, pp. 26–55.

Ferro-Luzzi, Gabriella Eichinger, 'Food Avoidances of Indian Tribes', *Anthropos*, Bd. 70, H. 3./4., 1975, pp. 385–427.

Foster, George M., 'Disease Etiologies in Non-Western Medical Systems', *American Anthropologists*, New Series, vol. 78, no. 4, 1976, pp. 773–82.

Furer-Haimendorf, Christoph von, 'Pre-Buddhist Elements in Sherpa Belief and Ritual', *Man*, vol. 55, April 1955, pp. 49–52.

Furer-Haimendorf, Christoph von, 'Religious Beliefs and Rituals of the Minyong Abors of Assam, India', *Anthropos*, Bd. 49, H. 3/4., 1954, pp. 588–604.

Furer-Haimendorf, Christoph von, 'The Presidential Address-1976', *RAIN*, no. 18, February 1977, pp. 6–11.

Gangwar, A.K. and P.S. Ramakrishnan, 'Ethnobiological Notes on Some Tribes of Arunachal Pradesh, Northeastern India', *Economic Botany*, vol. 44, no. 1, 1990, pp. 94–105.

Garret, Frances, 'Critical Methods in Tibetan Medical Histories', *The Journal of Asian Studies*, vol. 66, no. 2, 2007, pp. 363–87.

Goswami, Pranjiv et al., 'Traditional healthcare Pratices among the Tagin tribes of Arunachal Pradesh', *Indian Journal of Traditional Knowledge*, vol. 8, no. 1, January 2009, pp. 127–30.

Guha, Ramachandra, 'Centering the Peripheral', *Hindustan Times*, 29 April 2008. Retrieved from: http://www.hindustantimes.com/StoryPage/Print/307763.aspx, accessed on 13 July 2017.

Guyot-Rechard, Berenice, 'Tour Diaries and Itinerant Governance in the Eastern Himalayas, 1909–1962', *The Historical Journal*, Cambridge University Press, 2017, pp. 1–24. Retrieved from https://www.cambridge.org/core, accessed 13 July 2017.

Hardiman, David, 'Knowledge of the Bhils and Their System of Healing', *The Indian Historical Review*, vol. XXXIII, no. 1, January 2006, pp. 202–24.

Hilaly, Sarah, 'Representation of the Ethnic Communities of North-East: An Overview', *Proceedings of the North East India History Association*, Dibrugarh, 2008, pp. 415–19.

Hilaly, Sarah, 'Trajectory of Region Formation in the Eastern Himalayas', *Indian Historical Review*, vol. 42, no. 2, 2015, pp. 288–302.

Huber, Toni, 'Descent, Tutelaries and Ancestors, Transmission among Autonomous, *Bon* Ritual Specialist in Eastern Bhutan and the Mon-yul Corridor', in *From Bhakti to Bon*, ed. Hanna Havnevik and Charles Ramble, Oslo: Novus Press, 2015, pp. 271–90.

Jones, Rex L., 'Shamanism in South Asia: A Preliminary Survey', *History of Religions*, vol. 7, no. 4, May 1968, pp. 330–47.

Keenleyside, Anne, 'Changing Patterns of Health and Disease among the Aleuts', *Arctic Anthropology*, vol. 40, no. 1, 2003, pp. 48–69.

Kejriwal, O.P., 'The North-East in Indian Historiography: The Need for a Corrective', *Proceedings of the North East India History Association*, 7th Session, Pasighat, 1986, pp. 17–24.

Kingdon-Ward, Frank, 'Aftermath of the Great Assam Earthquake of 1950', *The Geographical Journal*, vol. 121, no. 3, September 1955, pp. 290–303.

Kvaerne, Per, 'Bon and Shamanism', *East and West*, vol. 59. nos. 1–4, 2009, pp. 19–24.

Lahariya, Chandrakant, 'A Brief History of Vaccines &Vaccination in India', *Indian Journal of Medical Research*, vol. 139, no. 4, April 2014, pp. 491–511.

Luthra, P.N., 'North-East Frontier Agency Tribes: Impact of Ahom and British Policy', *Economic and Political Weekly*, vol. 6, no. 23, 5 June 1971, pp. 1143–5, 1147–9.

Macfarlane, Alan and Mark Turin, 'Obituary: Professor Christoph von Fürer-Haimendorf 1909–1995', *Bulletin of the School of Oriental and African Studies, University of London*, vol. 59, no. 3, 1996, pp. 548–51.

Mandal, Pratyusa Kumar, 'Perspectives on Modernisation: Review of Select Researches Done on Arunachal Pradesh', *Proceedings of the*

North East India History Association, 20th Session, Dibrugarh, 2000, pp. 290–9.

Mathez-Stiefel, Sarah-Lan, Ina Vandebroek, and Stephan Rist, 'Can Andean Medicine Coexist with Biomedical Healthcare? A Comparison of Two Rural Communities in Peru and Bolivia', *Journal of Ethnobiology and Ethnomedicine*, vol. 8, no. 26, 2012, pp. 1–14.

Mills, J.P., 'The Mishmis of the Lohit Valley, Assam', *The Journal of Royal Anthropological Institute of Great Britain and Ireland*, vol. 82, no. 1, January–June 1952, pp. 1–12.

Mipun, B.S. and Debendrak Nayak, 'A Geographical Background to Peopling of North-East India: A Study in the Dynamics of Identity and Inter-group Relations', in *Dynamics of Identity and Inter-group Relations*, ed. Kailash S. Aggarwal, Shimla: Indian Institute of Advanced Studies, 1999, pp. 17–28.

Momin, Mignonette, 'Generalization in Constructing Histories of North East India', *Proceedings of NEIHA*, 24th Session, Guwahati, 2003, pp. 32–44.

Morgan, Lynn M., 'Dependency Theory in the Political Economy of Health: An Anthropological Critique', *Medical Anthropology Quarterly, New Series*, vol. 1, no. 2, June 1987, pp. 131–54.

Namsa, Nima D. et al., 'Ethnobotany of the Monpa ethnic group at Arunachal Pradesh, India', *Journal of Ethnobiology and Ethnomedicine*, vol. 7, no. 14, October 2011, pp. 7–31.

Nayak, Prasanta Kumar, 'History of Arunachal Pradesh: Problem of Periodization', *Proceedings of the North East India History Association*, 28th Session, Goalpara, 2007, pp. 46–56.

Nimachow, Gibji, 'Sacred Places, Beliefs, Festivals and Rituals of the Aka of Palizi Village', in *Dynamics of Tribal Villages in Arunachal Pradesh: Emerging Realities*, ed. Tamo Mibang and M.C. Behera, New Delhi: Mittal Publications, 2004, pp. 219–25.

Nishimura, Kho, 'Shamanism and Medical Cures', *Current Anthropology*, vol. 28, no. 4, Supplement: An Anthropological Profile of Japan, August–October 1987, pp. 59–64.

Panda, S., 'Fresh Dimensions to the Study of the British Relationship with the Tribes of Arunachal Pradesh', *Proceedings of the North*

East India History Association, 8th Session, Kohima, 1987, pp. 428–34.

Pavlik, Steve, 'Navajo Christianity: Historical Origins and Modern Trends', *Wicazo Sa Review*, vol. 12, no. 2, 1997, pp. 43–58.

Prasad, R.N., 'Inner Line Regulation and its Impact on Development of North-Eastern States', in *India's North-East-The Process of Change and Development*, ed. R.K. Samanta, Delhi: B.R. Publishing Corp., 1994, pp. 89–114.

Radhakrishnan, Meena, 'Of Apes and Ancestors: Evolutionary Science and Colonial Ethnogrpahy', *The Indian Historical Review*, vol. XXXIII, no. 1, Jan. 2006, pp. 1–23.

Ray, B. Datta, 'An aspect of the North East Frontier Policy of the Raj: An Overview', *Proceedings ofthe North East India History Association*, 6th Session, Agartala, 1985, pp. 226–9.

Reeve, Mary-Elizabeth, 'Concept of Illness and Treatment Practice in a Cabolo Community of the Lower Amazon', *Medical Anthropology Quarterly*, New Series, vol. 14, no. 1, March 2000, pp. 96–108.

Romero-Daza, Nancy, 'Traditional Medicine in Africa', *Annals of the American Academy of Political and Social Science*, vol. 583, Global Perspectives on Complementary and Alternative Medicine, September 2002, pp. 173–6.

Roolf, Becka, 'Healing Objects in Welsh Folk Medicine', *Proceedings of the Harvard Celtic Colloquim*, vols. 16/17, 1996/1997.

Sangma, Milton, 'Attempts to Christianize the People of Arunachal by the American Baptist missionaries (1836–1950)', *Proceedings of the North East India History Association*, 7th Session, Pasighat, 1980, pp. 263–72.

Schlesinger, Rudolf, 'Recent Discussions on the Periodization of History', *Soviet Studies*, vol. 4, no. 2, October 1952, pp. 152–69.

Shakspo, Nawang Tsering, 'Tibetan (Bhoti)—An Endangered Script in Trans-Himalaya',*The Tibet Journal*, vol. 30, no. 1, Spring 2005, pp. 61–4.

Showren, Tana, 'Ethnohistory in Arunachal Pradesh: Difficulties and Scope', *Proceedings of the North East India History Association*, 27th Session, Aizawl, 2006, pp. 46–54.

Sikdar, Sudatta, 'Cross-Country Trade in the Making of British Policy

Towards Arunachalis in the Nineteenth Century', *Proceedings of the North East India History Association*, 2nd Session, Dibrugarh, 1981, pp. 210–24.

Sikdar, Sudatta, 'Tribalism vs. Colonialism: British Capitalistic Intervention and Transformation of Primitive Economy of Arunachal Pradesh in the Nineteenth Century', *Social Scientist*, vol. 10, no. 12, December 1982, pp. 15–31.

Stonor, Charles, R., 'Notes on the Religion and Rituals of the Dafla Tribes of the Assam Himalayas', *Anthropos*, Bd. 52, H. 1/2. 1957, pp. 1–23.

Syiemlieh, David R., Presidential Address, *Proceedings of the North East India History Association*, 31st Session, Tura, 2010, pp. 1–15.

Taylor, Betsy, 'Public Folklore, Nation-Building, and Regional Others: Comparing Appalachian USA and North-East India', *Indian Folklore Research Journal,* vol. 1, no. 2, 2002, pp. 1–27.

Thakur, Amrendra Kumar, 'Peasantisation and State Formation in Early Arunachal Pradesh', *Proceedings of the Indian History Congress,* 58th Session, 1997, pp. 303–12.

Thakur, Amrendra Kumar, 'Processes and Agency of Precolonial States in Arunachal Pradesh,' *The NEHU Journal of Social Sciences and Humanities*, vol. 1, no. 1, January 2003, pp. 1–25.

Thakur, Amrendra Kumar, 'Social Transition in Pre-Colonial Arunachal Pradesh: Servitude as a Prime Mover', *Proceedings of the Indian History Congress,* 60th Session, 1999, pp. 391–403.

Thakur, Amrendra Kumar, 'Socio-Economic Formations in Pre-Colonial Arunachal: Myth and Reality', *The Indian Historical Review,* vol. XXXII, no. 2, July 2005, pp. 37–63.

Thakur, Amrendra Kumar, 'State Formation in Arunachal Pradesh', *The NEHU Journal of Social Sciences and Humanities*, vol. 1, no. 1, 1998, pp. 73–87.

Thupten (Shakya), Ngawang, 'Sowa-Rigpa: Affordable and Effective Traditional System of Tibetan/Himalayan Medicine for the People of Arunachal Pradesh', in *Tribal Development and Northeast India*, ed. Hage Lasa et al., New Delhi: Adhyayan Publishers and Distributors, 2013, pp. 142–58.

Waldram, James, B., 'The Efficacy of Traditional Medicine: Current

Theoretical and Methodological Issues', *Medical Anthropology Quarterly*, New Series, vol. 14, no. 4, 2000, pp. 603–25.

Walsh, E.H.C., 'Tibetan Anatomical System', *Journal of the Royal Asiatic Society of Great Britain and Ireland*, October 1910, pp. 1215–45.

Wardlow, Holly, 'Giving Birth to Gonolia: "Culture" and Sexually Transmitted Disease among the Huli of Papua New Guinea', *Medical Anthropology Quarterly*, New Series, vol. 16, no. 2, June 2002, pp. 151–75.

Wouters, Jelle J.P. and Tanka B. Subba, 'The "Indian Face", India's Northeast, and "The Idea of India"', *Asian Anthropology*, vol. 12, no. 2, 2013, pp. 126–40.

Books

Allen, B.C. et al., *Gazetteer of Bengal and North-East India*, 1905; repr., New Delhi: Mittal Publication, 2012.

Arnold, David, *Colonizing the Body: State, Medicine and Epidemic Diseases in Nineteenth-century India*, Berkley: University of California Press, 1993.

Arnold, David, ed., *Imperial Medicine and Indigenous Societies*, New York: Manchester University Press, 1988.

Bala, Poonam, *Imperialism and Medicine in Bengal: A Socio-Historical Perspective*, New Delhi: Sage Publications, 1991.

Bannerjee, Bikash, *The Bokars: An Anthropological Research on their Ecological Settings and Social Systems*, Itanagar: Directorate of Research, Government of Arunachal Pradesh, 1999.

Barpujari, H.K., *American Baptist Missionaries and North East India, 1836–1900: A Documentary Study*,Gauhati: Spectrum Publications, 1986.

———, *Problem of Hill Tribes: North East Frontier 1822–42*, vol. I, Gauhati: Lawyer's Book Stall, 1970.

Barua, Sanjib, *India Against Itself: Assam and the Politics of Nationality*, New Delhi: Oxford University Press, 1999.

Baruah, Tapan Kumar M., *The Idu Mishmis*, Itanagar: Directorate of Research, Government of Arunachal Pradesh, 1960.

Bibliography

Bhadra, R.K. and Mita Bhadra, eds., *Ethnicity, Movement and Social Structure: Contested Cultural Identity*, New Delhi: Rawat Publication, 2007.

Bhattacharjee, Tarun Kumar, *Alluring Frontiers*, Gauhati: Omsons Publications, 1987.

———, *Enticing Frontiers*, New Delhi: Omsons Publications, 1992.

———, *The Frontier Trail*, Calcutta: Manick Bandhopadhyay, 1993.

———, *The Idus of Dree and Mathun Valley*, Itanagar: Directorate of Research, Government of Arunachal Pradesh, 1983.

Blackburn, Stuart, *Into the Hidden Valley: A Novel*, New Delhi: Speaking Tiger, 2016.

———, *The Sun Rises. A Shaman's Chant, Ritual Exchange and Fertility in the Apatani Valley*, Leiden: Brill (Brill's Tibetan Studies Library, 16/3), 2010.

Boban, K. Jose, *Tribal Ethnomedicine: Continuity and Change*, New Delhi: APH Publishing Corp., 1998.

Bordoloi, Chandra, *Call of the Blue Hills: Recollections from Arunachal Pradesh*, New Delhi: National Book Trust, 2012.

Boruah, Nirode, *Historical Geography of Early Assam*, Guwahati: DVS Publisher, 2010.

Bose, M.L., *History of Arunachal Pradesh*, New Delhi: Concept Publishing, 1977.

Bose, Nirmal Kumar, *The Structure of Hindu Society*, tr. Andre Beteille, 3rd revd edn, Hyderabad: Orient Longman, 1994.

Bower, Ursula Graham, *The Hidden Land: Mission to a Far Corner of India*, New York: William Morrow & Company, 1953.

Butler, John, *A Sketch of Assam: With Some Accounts of the Hills Tribes*, London: Smith, Elder & Co., 1847.

———, *Travels and Adventures in the Province of Assam, during a Residence of Fourteen Years*, London: Smith, Elder & Co., 1855.

Cederlof, Gunnel, *Founding an Empire on India's North-Eastern Frontiers 1790–1840: Climate, Commerce, Polity*, New Delhi: Oxford University Press, 2014.

Chakravarty, L.N., *Glimpses of the Early History of Arunachal*, Itanagar: Government of Arunachal Pradesh, 1995.

Chaliha, Parag, ed., *The Outlook on NEFA*, Jorhat: Asam Sahitya Sabha, 1958.

Chari, Chandra and Uma Iyengar, eds., *The Public Intellectual in India*, New Delhi: Aleph Book, 2015.

Chaube, S.K., *Hill Politics in Northeast India*, 3rd revd edn, New Delhi: Orient BlackSwan, 2012.

Childe, Gordon, *What Happened in History*, Middlesex, USA: Penguin Books, 1957.

Choudhury, S. Dutta, ed., *Gazetteer of India: Arunachal Pradesh: East and West Siang Districts*, Shillong: Government of Arunachal Pradesh, 1994.

———, ed., *Gazetteer of India: Arunachal Pradesh: East Kameng, West Kameng and Tawang Districts*, Shillong: Government of Arunachal Pradesh, 1996.

———, ed., *Gazetteer of India: Arunachal Pradesh: Lohit District*, Itanagar: Government of Arunachal Pradesh, 2008.

———, ed., *Gazetteer of India: Arunachal Pradesh: Subansiri District*, Itanagar: Government of Arunachal Pradesh, 2008.

———, ed., *Gazetteer of India: Arunachal Pradesh: Tirap District*, Itanagar: Government of Arunachal Pradesh, 2008.

———, ed., *Gazetteer of India: Arunachal Pradesh: State Gazetteer of Arunachal Pradesh*, vol. I, Itanagar: Government of Arunachal Pradesh, 2010.

Curtin, Phillip D., *Death by Migration: Europe's Encounter with the Tropical World in the Nineteenth Century*, New York: Cambridge University Press, 1989.

Dalton, E.T., *Descriptive Ethnology of Bengal*, Calcutta: Office of the Superintendent of Government Printing, 1872.

Darwin, John, *The Empire Project: The Rise and Fall of the British World-System, 1830–1970*, New York: Cambridge University Press, 2009.

Das, B.M., *The Peoples of Assam*, Delhi: Gian Publishing House, 1987.

Das, Durga, *India from Curzon to Nehru and After*, New Delhi: Rupa, 2015.

Dawar, Jagdish Lal, *Cultural Identity of Tribes of North-East India:*

Movement for Cultural Identity Among the Adis of Arunachal Pradesh, New Delhi: Commonwealth Publishers, 2003.

Deuri, R.K., *The Sulungs,* Itanagar: Directorate of Research, Government of Arunachal Pradesh, 1982.

Devi, Lakshmi, *Ahom-Tribal Relations: A Political Study,* Gauhati: Assam Book Depot, 1968.

Downs, Frederick S., *History of Christianity in India*, vol. V, part 5, Bangalore: The Church History Association of India, 2003.

Duff-Sutherland-Dunbar, George, *Other Men's Lives: A Study of Primitive Peoples*, London: The Scientific Book Club, 1938.

Dutta, Parul, *Aspects of Padam Minyong Culture,* 2nd edn, Itanagar: Government of Arunachal Pradesh, 1966.

———, *The Tangsas,* Itanagar: Directorate of Research, Government of Arunachal Pradesh, 2010.

Dutta, S. and B. Tripathy, *Sources of the History of Arunachal Pradesh*, New Delhi: Gyan Publishing House, 2008.

Elwin, Verrier, *A Philosophy for NEFA*, 1957; repr., Itanagar: Government of Arunachal Pradesh, 2006.

———, *Democracy in NEFA*, 1965; repr., Itanagar: Government of Arunachal Pradesh, 2007.

———, ed. and comp., *India's North East Frontier in the Nineteenth Century*, Bombay: Oxford University Press, 1959.

———, *Myths of the North-East Frontier of India*, 1958; repr., New Delhi: Munshiram Manoharlal, 1999.

———, *The Art of the North-East Frontier of India*, 1959; repr., Itanagar: Government of Arunachal Pradesh, 2009.

Furer-Haimendorf, Christoph von, *A Himalayan Tribe: from Cattle to Cash*, Berkley: University of California Press, 1980.

———, *Highlanders of Arunachal Pradesh*, New Delhi: Vikas Publishing House, 1982.

———, *Himalayan Barbary*, 1955; repr., as *Himalayan Adventure*, New Delhi: Vikas Publishing House, 1983.

———, *The Apatanis and their Neighbours: A Primitive Civilisation of the Eastern Himalayas*, London: Routledge & Kegan Paul, 1962.

Gait, Edward, *A History of Assam*, 2nd edn, 1926; repr., Delhi: Surjeet Publications, 2004.

Goswami, Priyam, *The History of Assam: From Yandabo to Partition, 1826–1947*, New Delhi: Orient BlackSwan, 2012.

Gottlob, Michael, *History and Politics in Post-colonial India*, New Delhi: Oxford University Press, 2011.

Guha, Amalendu, *Planter Raj to Swaraj: Freedom Struggle and Electoral Politics in Assam, 1826–1947*, New Delhi: Tulika Books, 2006.

Guha, Ramachandra, *Democrats and Dissenters*, Gurgaon: Penguin Random House, 2016.

———, *India after Gandhi: The History of the World's Largest Democracy*, London: Picador India, 2008.

———, *Savaging the Civilized: Verrier Elwin, His Tribals, and India*, New Delhi: Oxford University Press, 2000.

Guyot-Rechard, Berenice, *Shadow States: India, China and the Himalayas, 1910–1962*, Cambridge: Cambridge University Press, 2017.

Haldipur, Krishna, *Around the Hills and Dales of Arunachal Pradesh*, Shillong: North Eastern Hill Univeristy, 1985.

Hamilton, Agnus, *In Abor Jungles of North East India*, 1912; repr., New Delhi: Mittal Publications, 2003. (Originally published as *In Abor Jungles: Being an Account of the Abor Expedition, the MishmiMission and the Miri Mission*, London: Eveleigh Nash, 1912).

Hardiman, David, *Missionaries and their Medicine: A Christian Modernity for Tribal India*, Manchester and NY: Manchester University Press, 2014.

Headrick, D.R., *The Tools of Empire: Technology and European Imperialism in the Nineteenth Century*, New York: Oxford University Press, 1981.

Hunter, W.W., *Statistical Account of Assam*, vol. I, London: Trübner & Co., 1879.

Hutton, J.H., *The Angami Nagas: With Some Notes on Some Neighbouring Tribes*, London: Macmillan & Co., 1921.

———, *The Sema Nagas*, London: Macmillan & Co., 1921.

Izzard, Ralph, *The Hunt for the Buru*: *The True Story of the Search for a Prehistoric Reptile in North India*, 1951; repr., California: Linden Publishing Inc., 2001.

Kaul, P.N., *Frontier Callings*, Delhi: Vikas Publishing House, 1976.

Kaviraj, Sudipta, *The Unhappy Consciousness: Bankimchandra Chattopad-*

hyay and the Formation of Nationalist Discourse in India, Delhi: Oxford University Press, 1995.

Kelm, Mary-Ellen, *Colonizing Bodies: Aboriginal Health and Healing in British Columbia, 1900–50*, Vancouver: UBC Press, 1998.

Kingdon-Ward, Frank, *Himalayan Enchantment: An Anthology*, London: Serinda Publications, 1990.

Krishnatry, S.M., *Border Tagins of Arunachal Pradesh*, New Delhi: National Book Trust, 2004.

Kumar, Anil, *Medicine and the Raj*, New Delhi: Sage Publication, 1998.

Kumar, Deepak, *Science and the Raj, 1857–1905*, Delhi: Oxford University Press, 1995.

———, ed., *Disease and Medicine in India: A Historical Overview*, New Delhi: Tulika Books, 2001.

Lake, Medicine Grizzlybear, *Native Healer: Initiation into an Ancient Art*, Illinois: Wheaton, 2007.

Leod, Roy Mac and Lewis Milton, eds., *Disease, Medicine and Empire: Perspectives of Western Medicine and the Experience of European Expansion*, London and NY: Routledge, 1988.

Leslie, Charles, ed., *Asian Medical System: A Comparative Study*, California: University of California Press, 1977.

Lobo, Lancy, *Malaria in the Social Context: A Study of Western India*, New Delhi and Abingdon (UK): Routledge, 2010.

Ludden, David, *India and South Asia: A Short History*, Oxford: Oneworld Publications, 2006.

Luthra, P.N., *Constitutional and Administrative Growth of the Arunachal Pradesh*, Shillong: North-East Frontier Agency, 1971.

M'Cosh, John, *Topography of Assam*, 1837; repr., New Delhi: Logos Press, 2000.

Mackenzie, Alexander, *The North East Frontier of India*, 1884; repr., New Delhi: Mittal Publication, 2004.

Mandelbaum, David G., *Society in India: I Continuity and Change, II Change and Continuity*, Mumbai: Popular Prakashan, 2011.

May, Andrew J., *Welsh Missionaries and British Imperialism: The Empire of Clouds in Northeast India*, Manchester: Manchester University Press, 2016.

Mibang, Tamo and S.K. Chaudhuri, eds., *Ethnomedicines of the Tribes of Arunachal Pradesh*, New Delhi: Himalayan Publishers, 2003.

Miller, Barbara D., *Cultural Anthropology*, 7th edn, New York: Pearson Education, 2012.

Mills, J.P., *The Rengma Nagas*, London: Macmillan & Co., 1937.

Mukherjee, Sujata, *Gender, Medicine, and Society in Colonial India: Women's Health Care in Nineteenth- and Early Twentieth-Century Bengal*, New Delhi: Oxford University Press, 2017.

Nag, Sajal, *Beleaguered Nation: The Making and Unmaking of the Assamese Nationality*, New Delhi: Manohar Publishers, 2017.

Nyori, Tai, *History and Culture of the Adis*, New Delhi: Omsons Publications, 1993.

Osik, N.N., *British Relations with the Adis (1825–1947)*, New Delhi: Omsons Publications, 1992.

Palit, Chittabrata and Achintya Dutta, eds., *History of Medicine in India: The Medical Encounter*, Delhi: Kalpaz Publications, 2011.

Pati, Biswamoy and Mark Harrison, eds., *Health, Medicine and Empire: Perspectives on Colonial on Colonial*, New Delhi: Orient Longman, 2001.

———, eds., *The Social History of Health and Medicine in Colonial India*, Delhi: Primus Books, 2013.

Pemberton, Robert Boileau, *The Eastern Frontier of India*, 1835; repr., New Delhi: Mittal Publications, 2015.

Pertin, Onyok, *Adi Among Sim Milun E' Aabomdak Dooying* ('The Story of Coming of the British in Adi Area'), Pasighat: Oming Pertin, 2014.

Reid, Robert, *History of Frontier Areas Bordering on Assam from 1883–1941*, 1942; repr., Delhi: Eastern Publishing House, 1983.

Riddi, Ashan, *The Tagins of Arunachal Pradesh: A Study of Continuity and Change*, Delhi: Abhijeet Publication, 2006.

Robinson, William, *Descriptive Account of Assam*, 1841; repr., Delhi: Sanskaran Prakashan, 1975.

Roy, Babul, *Medical Anthropology: Studies in the Highlands of Assam*, New Delhi: Serials Publications, 2012.

Rustomji, Nari, *Enchanted Frontiers: Sikkim, Bhutan and India's*

North-Eastern Borderlands, New Delhi: Oxford University Press, 2010.

Saikia, Pahi, *Ethnic Mobilisation and Violence in Northeast India*, New Delhi: Routledge, 2011.

Sangma, Milton, *History of American Baptist Mission in North East India*, vol. 1, New Delhi: Mittal Publications, 1996.

Scott, James C., *The Art of Not Being Governed: An Anarchist History of Upland Southeast Asia*, New Haven and London: Yale University Press, 2009.

Shakespear, L.W., *History of the Assam Rifles*, 1929; repr., Sussex, England: Naval and Military Press, 2005.

Shakespear, L.W., *History of Upper Assam, Upper Burmah and North-Eastern Frontier*, London: Macmillan & Co., 1914.

Shankar, Rama and M.S. Rawat, *Medico-Ethno-Botany of Arunachal Pradesh*, Itanagar: Regional Research Institute, AYUSH Regional Centre, 2008.

Sharma, Hirendra Nath, *Traditional Medicines of Arunachal Pradesh and Assam: Practice & Prospect*, Gauhati: Ashok Km Sharma, 2007.

Showren, Tana, *The Nyishi of Arunachal Pradesh: An Ethnohistorical Study*, New Delhi: Regency Publications, 2009.

Singh, K.S., ed., *People of India: Arunachal Pradesh*, vol. XIV, Calcutta: Anthropological Survey of India/Seagull Books, 1995.

Singh, Sudhir Kumar and Ashan Riddi, eds., *Pre-Colonial History and Traditions of Arunachal Pradesh*, Guwahati: DVS Publishers, 2017.

Srivastav, L.R.N., *Among the Wanchos*, 1970; repr., Itanagar: Directorate of Research, Government of Arunachal Pradesh, 2010.

———, *The Gallongs*, 1962; repr., Itanagar: Directorate of Research, Government of Arunachal Pradesh, 1988.

Syiemlieh, David R., ed., *On the Edge of Empire: Four British Plans for North East India, 1941–1947*, New Delhi: Sage Publications, 2014.

Tarr, Michael Aram and Stuart Blackburn, *Through the Eyes of Time: Photographs of Arunachal Pradesh, 1859–2006: Tribal Cultures in Eastern Himalayas*, Leiden and Boston: Brill, 2008.

Thakur, Amrendra Kumar, *Slavery in Arunachal Pradesh*, New Delhi: Mittal Publications, 2003.

Webster, John C.B., *Historiography of Christianity in India*, New Delhi: Oxford University Press, 2012.

Government Reports

Arunachal Pradesh Human Development Report, 2005, Itanagar: Department of Planning, Government of Arunachal Pradesh, 2006.

Census of India 1971: Series-24, Arunachal Pradesh, Part-VIII-A: Administration Report – Enumeration.

Census of India, 1961: Volume XXIV: North East Frontier Agency, Part II-A, General Population Tables and NEFA Special Tables.

Census of India: Demographic and Socio-economic Profiles of the Hill Areas of North East India, Office of the Registrar General, India, Ministry of Home Affairs, New Delhi, 1970.

Census, 1951: Assam: North East Frontier Agency District Census Handbook.

Economic Review of Arunachal Pradesh, 1988, Shillong: Directorate of Economics and Statistics, Government of Arunachal Pradesh.

International Council on Archives: Guide to the Sources of Asian History, India 3.2, New Delhi: National Archives of India, 1992.

Statistical Abstract, 1988, Arunachal Pradesh, Shillong: Directorate of Economics and Statistics, Government of Arunachal Pradesh.

Statistical Atlas of Arunachal Pradesh, 1995, Itanagar: Directorate of Economics and Statistics, Government of Arunachal Pradesh.

Statistical Outline of North East Frontier Agency, April 1958, Shillong: Directorate of Economics and Statistics, Government of Arunachal Pradesh.

Statistical Outline of North East Frontier Agency, April 1960, Shillong: The Statistical Branch, NEFA.

Statistical Outline of North East Frontier Agency, April 1961, Shillong: The Statistical Branch, NEFA.

Statistical Outline of North East Frontier Agency, April 1963, Shillong: The Statistical Branch, NEFA.

Statistical Outline of North East Frontier Agency, April 1966, Shillong: The Statistical Department, NEFA.

Statistical Outline of North East Frontier Agency, April 1967, Shillong: The Statistical Department, NEFA.

Techno-Economic Survey of NEFA: Economic Report, New Delhi: National Council of Applied Economic Research, December 1965 (MS, State Research Library, Government of Arunachal Pradesh, Itanagar).

Online Sources

http://blog.cpsindia.org/2016/02/religion-data-of-census-2011-xiii.htmlhttp://www.census2011.co.in/census/state/arunachal+pradesh.html

http://www.arunachalpradesh.gov.in/bio.htm

http://www.hindustantimes.com/StoryPage/Print/307763.aspx

http://www.jstor.org

Oral Sources

Interviews by the Author

Guru Tulku Rinpoche (Abbot, Gaden Namgyal Lhatse, Tawang Monastery). 15 April 2015, Tawang, Arunachal Pradesh.

Wangdi Lama (Khinmey Monastery (Nyigmapa), Tawang). 15 April 2015, Tawang, Arunachal Pradesh.

Tsering Tobgey (herbal expert, Gomkhang Medicinal Garden, Gomkhang Village, Tawang). 16 April 2015, Tawang, Arunachal Pradesh.

Tama Mindo Romin (Shaman). 6 January 2017 A-Sector, Naharlagun, Arunachal Pradesh.

Tadar Nipo (son of Tadar Nyipo, Shaman). 7 January 2017, Doimukh, Papum Pare District, Arunachal Pradesh.

Bibliography

Un-Published Dissertations

Ibata, Atsuko, 'Community Mental Health and Folk Psychiatry in Tribal India', PhD diss., University of Delhi, 2014.

Jha, Braj Narain, 'British Colonial Intervention and Tribal Responses in the North EastFrontier of Assam, 1825–1947', PhD diss., Arunachal University, 2002.

Mene, Tarun, 'Suicide among the Idu Mishmi Tribe of Arunachal Pradesh', PhD diss., Rajiv Gandhi University, 2011.

Miso, Rajiv, 'Priesthood among the Idu-Mishmis', MPhil diss., Rajiv Gandhi University, 2005.

Naku, Hage, 'Beliefs and Practices of Apatanis—Study in Continuity and Change', PhD diss., Rajiv Gandhi University, 2006.

Rikam, Nabam Tadar, 'Changing Religious Identity of Arunachal Pradesh: A Case Study of the Nyishi since 1947', PhD diss., Arunachal University, 2003.

Yampi, Radhe, 'Religious Specialist of the Apatanis: Aspects of their Nature, Structure and Change', PhD diss., Rajiv Gandhi University, 2009.

Index

www.ingramcontent.com/pod-product-compliance
Lightning Source LLC
LaVergne TN
LVHW101915190826
846094LV00004B/60/J

* 9 7 8 9 3 5 6 8 7 0 4 4 4 *